Mindful
Chef

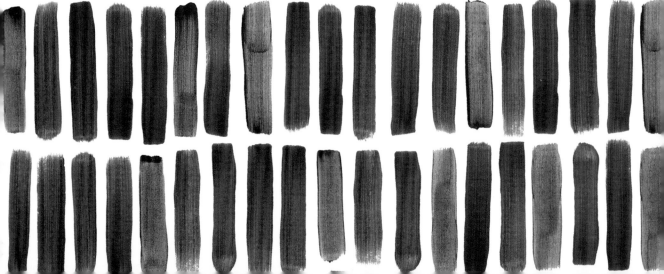

MYLES HOPPER + GILES HUMPHRIES

Mindful
Chef

30-minute meals to get lean, reduce stress,
increase energy levels and enjoy better sleep

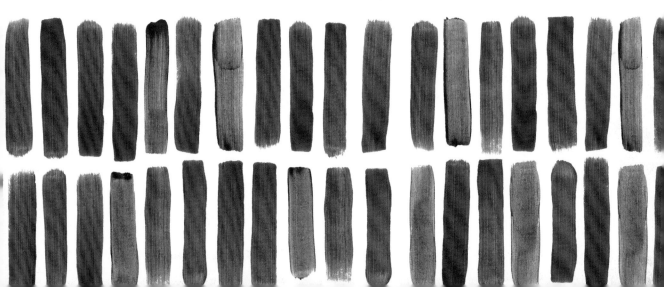

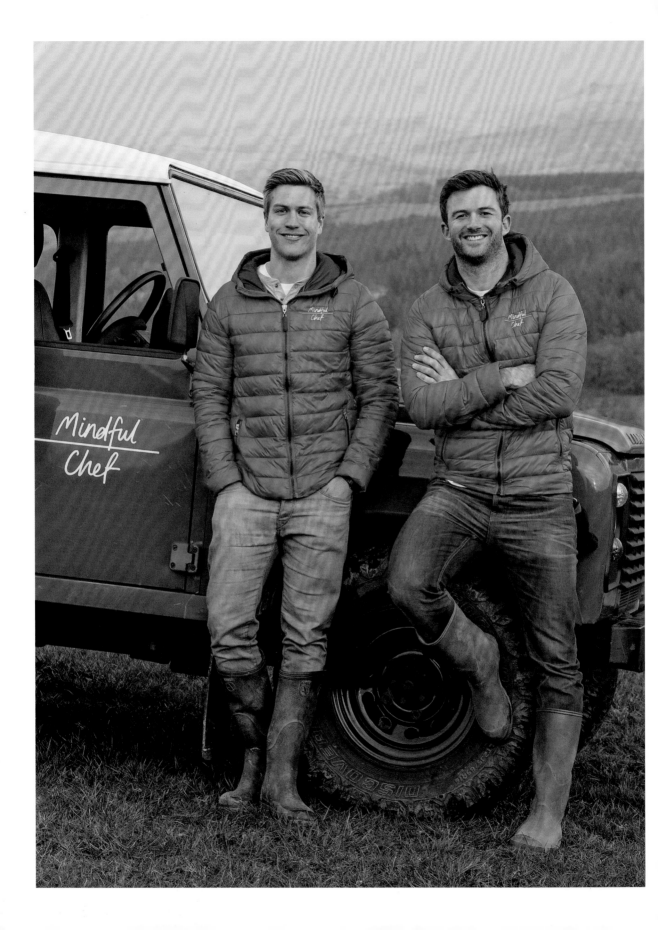

CONTENTS

INTRODUCTION

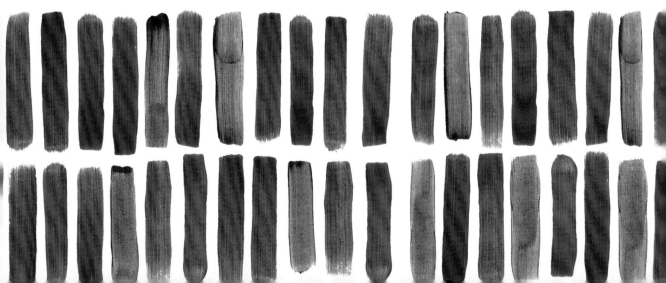

OUR STORY

It all began back in 1999 when Myles and I met at school in Exeter, Devon. Surrounded by the rugged Dartmoor National Park and the rolling hills of Devon, it was a wonderful place to grow up. We played a lot of sport and spent our weekends out and about enjoying the countryside, particularly the array of beautiful beaches that the West Country has to offer. The delicious local food, and it has to be said, the cider, were a huge part of our upbringing, too, and something that we soon realised we took for granted. Every year we would travel down with our families and spend the summer holidays on the Cornish beaches, not far from where we source our fresh fish today. We'd often hit the surf together before kicking back in the campsite around a campfire. Myles still claims he is a better surfer.

Fast-forward 17 years and we found ourselves in London; Myles was working as a nutritional coach and personal trainer and I was working at an advertising agency. We both had stable jobs and were enjoying ourselves, despite craving the West Country. However, we were working long hours and returning home late in the evenings, usually too knackered to cook a healthy meal. I would often settle for yet another pasta dish on repeat, or a quick ready-meal. Couple that with the usual sandwich at lunch and I was getting little to no nutritional balance in my diet. It doesn't take a rocket scientist to work out that you shouldn't eat McDonalds or Burger King every week, but a lot of people don't appreciate the harm they are doing to their bodies when the bulk of their daily intake is pasta and bread. Both are refined carbohydrates and possess little nutritional value. When you look around, it is no wonder we are in the middle of a health epidemic. In short, we weren't leading the lives we wanted to, and we realised that food was a big part of this. With Myles's background in nutrition, we knew how much food can affect mood, health and general well-being.

It was in early 2015 that we thought enough was enough, and decided to take the leap. We quit our jobs at the same time, and tried to find a solution. Over long coffees (with the occasional green tea) and late nights we drew up what we felt was the ideal answer for people craving a convenient way to eat well regularly. Mindful Chef – which would become the UK's favourite healthy recipe box company, delivering delicious recipes to thousands of customers each week – was born.

It was important for us that mindfulness sat right across everything we did from the outset. Why mindfulness? It's a word that is thrown around a lot

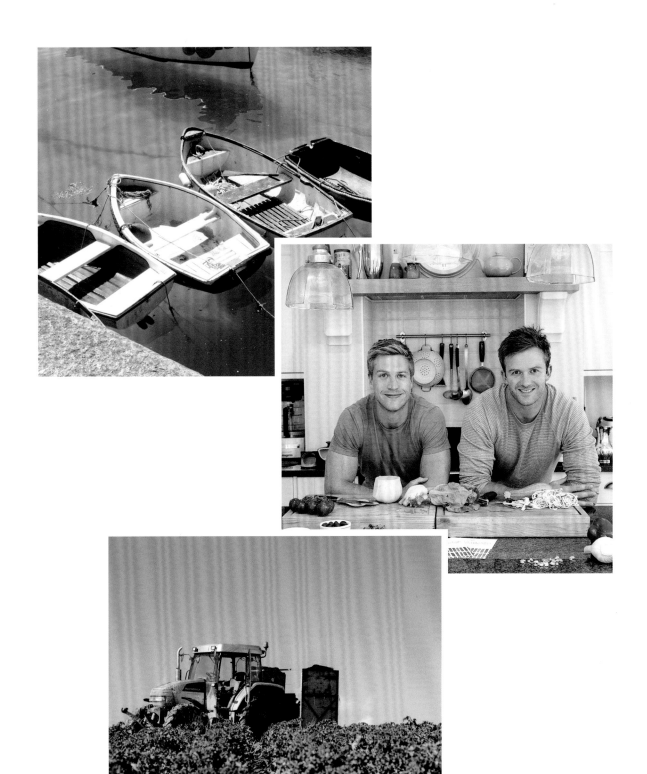

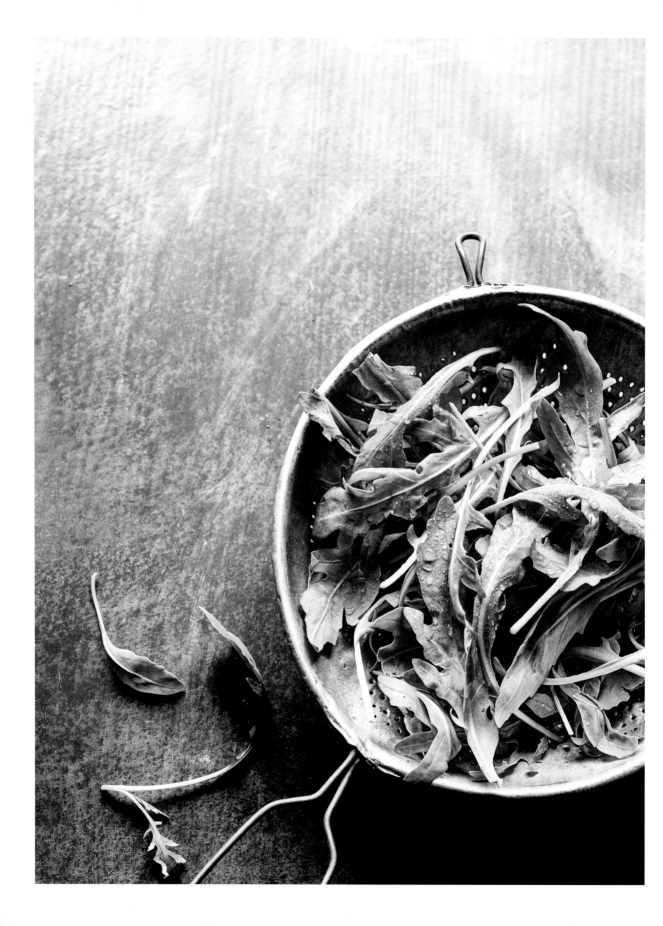

these days, but to us it simply means being conscious of the world around us, and of living in the present. We wanted to slow down from the hectic speed of city life. When it comes to living a healthy, fulfilling lifestyle, food and nutrition is a fundamental part of mindfulness. And we wanted to be mindful of the whole process, from bringing food fresh from farm to fork in as little time as possible (cutting out the supermarket middle men and bulky supply chains), of reducing food waste (we only deliver exactly the right amount of food so people don't throw away excess produce), right through to the very ingredients we choose to help people live a more balanced and energised life.

Working from my small flat in South London we combined long hours of recipe testing with trips to the West Country to meet as many suppliers as possible. It was incredibly important to us to bring our customers the best produce available direct from the farms and fishermen. Back and forth we went, searching high and low for the very highest-quality local produce. Some days we would be up at 5am meeting the fishermen on the docks at Penzance watching the boats land their catches, then we'd head up to Dartmoor for the afternoon to visit a host of farms nestled in the lush fertile Devon valleys. Life was busy but it was good; we felt like progress was being made and the more we saw of this quality of produce, the more we thought that we had to bring this way of eating to more people.

Equally as important was the type of recipes we created. Recipes had to be wholesome, contain absolutely no refined carbs, be 100 per cent gluten free and most importantly of all, be incredibly delicious. Early on, we found a helping hand in this department when we met Louisa, a professional chef, who would help us hone our skills in the kitchen and develop delicious recipes. Louisa trained at Leith's, the prestigious cookery school in London, and then went on to travel and gain experience cooking in Asia where she brought back some wonderful tips and tricks which go into our recipes every week. We don't profess to be professional chefs and to some extent that is the whole point of Mindful Chef. It is about bringing cooking back into the lives of people who may not have had the time or inclination to dive into the kitchen on a regular basis.

We started packing our first Mindful Chef boxes in my kitchen in April of 2015. Our first 10 customers were our loyal friends and families, most of whom still receive their box each week without fail. We would deliver our boxes of goodness in a small van emblazoned proudly with our new logo on the side; our little venture had become a reality.

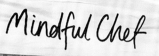
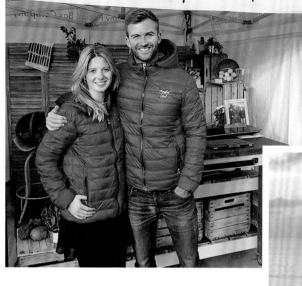
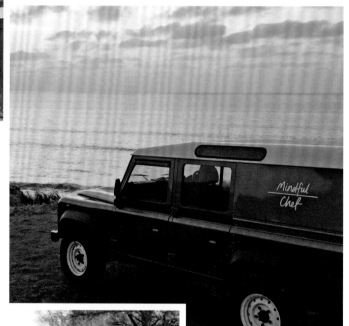
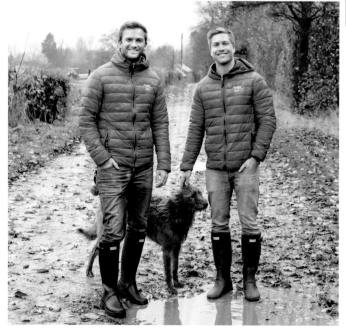

And here we find ourselves today. We now deliver to thousands of households across the country (with the help of some professional couriers, I might add). We have a fantastic team helping bring Mindful Chef to life and a loyal customer base who seem to love the recipes as much as we do.

We are extremely excited to bring you this book full of healthy, seasonal and – most importantly –delicious recipes. They are divided into five sections that will help you improve different areas of your life: energy and productivity; stress, gut health, exercise and sleep.

Each of our 70 recipes contains no more than eight steps and will take less than 30 minutes to cook from start to finish, nor do they require any food processors or expensive utensils. Most of our recipes contain no more than 10 ingredients. It is incredibly important to us that these meals genuinely are a convenient way to fit healthy eating into a busy modern lifestyle – you'll finish cooking each meal thinking 'that was easy'.

You can expect to come away from each meal feeling satisfied yet energised. The ingredients we use mean you won't feel that sugar high and then the inevitable slump. Your insulin levels will be balanced and your body filled with vitamins and nutrients so you'll have no need to rely on a strong coffee or a sugar-laden sandwich followed by that sticky mid-afternoon treat to get you through your day. Your body will thank you and as a result you will likely start making other mindful changes to your lifestyle.

Cooking up Mindful Chef recipes on a regular basis has visible health benefits. Our customers report sleeping better, being more productive, feeling stress-free, feeling leaner, having more focus, having clearer skin and generally feeling very good about themselves.

We hope you will enjoy eating the mindful way. There's no fasting, juicing or crash-dieting, you'll find yourself eating heaps of nutritious vegetables and fantastic, flavoursome natural produce. We don't believe in meticulous calorie counting or following strict diets; we simply want to encourage you to eat good, wholesome food that benefits you and your body.

PROVENANCE

These days it is difficult to know where your food comes from, how animals have been treated, or what chemicals have been sprayed on to the fresh produce you buy. It's for this reason we work with British farmers and producers, not only to support local businesses, but also to ensure complete traceability. We love getting out and meeting with our suppliers to talk to them about their farming methods and above all to guarantee they are practising the same mindful beliefs as us.

GREAT HEALTH STARTS WITH GREAT PRODUCE

We believe in ethical and sustainable farming and place great importance on the provenance of all of our produce. We know that people who care about their health and what they eat want to make informed and responsible choices. Like us these people don't want their food to be tampered with, chemically altered or changed in any way, but instead prefer to eat food in its natural form; and for the most part, want to know how it's been grown or reared.

The farmers and producers we work with adhere to the highest ethical farming standards and take responsibility for their impact on the environment. They use fewer pesticides and pay great attention to animal welfare. Consequently, the food they produce is rich in nutrients, which will have a positive effect on the processes our bodies carry out every day.

It's not always easy to trace the provenance of your food, but the most important thing you can do is ask questions: find out how it has been grown or reared. Choosing to buy organic food is one way of obtaining this kind of reassurance, but there are lots of farmers who don't have the official organic accreditation but who do still farm organically and in a sustainable and mindful way. Some of the smaller, local British farms we use simply cannot afford the Soil Association organic accreditation. Stephen at the British Quinoa Company is a fantastic example of someone who supplies quality produce that isn't organic but is grown using low input and sustainable production methods that are good for both the environment and you.

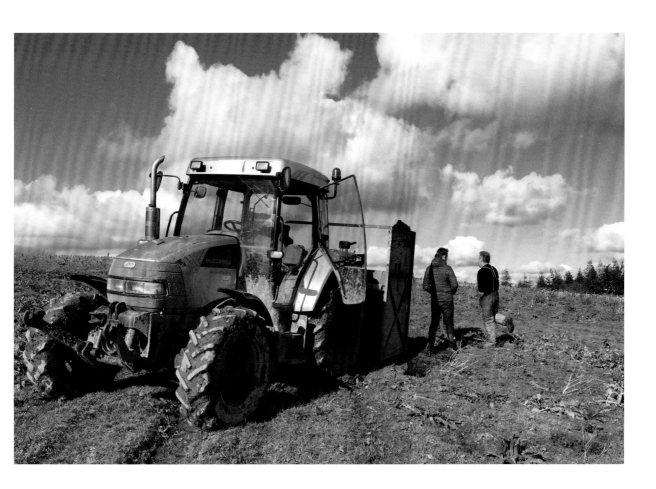

It was Farmer Govier from Langridge Organic Farm near where we grew up in the West Country who taught us about sustainable farming. Standing in the middle of a field of purple sprouting broccoli in Devon's rolling hills, he pointed at the farm. 'Those fields over there are in fallow. For three to four years, they are covered in grass and clover and sheep are brought in to graze. The sheep droppings put nitrates back into the soil – they're walking fertiliser dispensers!' Once Farmer Govier has farmed his field he has to leave that field for three years to allow the animals to restore the soil fertility naturally. Yet because Farmer Govier, who supplies us with spinach, sprouts, kale and other brassicas, doesn't use man-made fertilisers, there are no foreign chemicals on his land. Chemicals in fertilisers negatively interact with plants and reduce the formation of antioxidants, which are vital to the inner workings of your body, helping with everything from having great looking skin, to preventing premature ageing, to reducing the chances of developing heart disease or cancer.

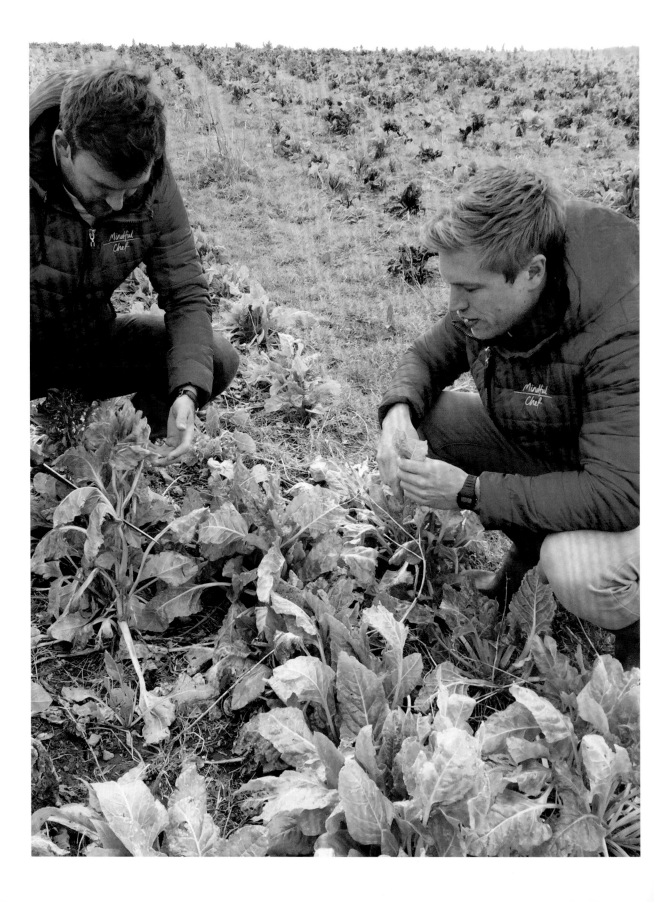

Outdoor-reared, grass-fed animals produce meat that is consistently higher in desirable omega-3 fatty acids than grain-fed beef

ANIMAL WELFARE

When it comes to our meat, we like to know what the animals have been eating for their entire lives. Nowadays, despite evolving to eat grass, and grass only, most farmed cattle are fed grain and cereals. This fattens them up quicker, resulting in less time in the field and more profit. Unfortunately, you pay for this in taste, tenderness and in the nutritional quality of the meat.

We believe livestock must have access to the outdoors. Outdoor-reared, grass-fed animals produce meat that is consistently higher in desirable omega-3 fatty acids than grain-fed beef – the fatty acids are essential for a healthy heart. They are also high in natural carotene (found in the grass) which is important for eye health. Mark Bury at Eversfield Organic, who supplies us with beef from his farm to the north of Dartmoor National Park in Devon, rears cattle which eat grass their entire life. Devon's rich soil and heavy rainfall means it has some of the finest grass in the country.

We also choose to source meat reared by farmers who are not using antibiotics. Livestock are often fed antibiotics to keep them from getting ill and growth hormones to encourage them to grow more quickly. Antibiotics that are fed to livestock end up entering our bodies and could easily have an impact on our own immune system's ability to defend itself, particularly in later life.

You have to ask yourself the question: would you rather eat animals that have been able to roam fields, or ones which are kept inside for most of their lives? Which would you rather eat and put into your body? Do you really want to eat a piece of meat that has come from an animal being fed antibiotics to keep it from being ill, or growth hormones to encourage it to grow quicker? It goes without saying that if you really care about your health you probably won't want to put these foreign substances into your body without knowing exactly the effects they might have on it.

MINDFUL FARMING

Mindful farming is about getting the most out of the soil and protecting the countryside's unique ecosystem. It strives for sustainability, better soil fertility and biological diversity without relying on any methods that may upset this fragile system, such as synthetic pesticides, antibiotics, fertilisers, growth hormones and genetically modified foods. Farming in this way has been proven to increase the biodiversity of species found on farms. Trees, rivers, hedgerows, insects, bees, flora and the animals that roam all contribute to the production of great food and ensure that we don't degrade our soil to the point that it dies. If you have chemicals on crops, or farms, they can harm insects and consequently other animals that may eat them.

We believe passionately in supporting local farmers who help protect Britain's great countryside and Mark from Eversfield Organic is another great example. Since taking over Eversfield, Mark has planted over 10,000 trees, rebuilt hedgerows and does not use any harmful chemicals on his land. His beautiful farm is a joy to visit and we get down there several times a year.

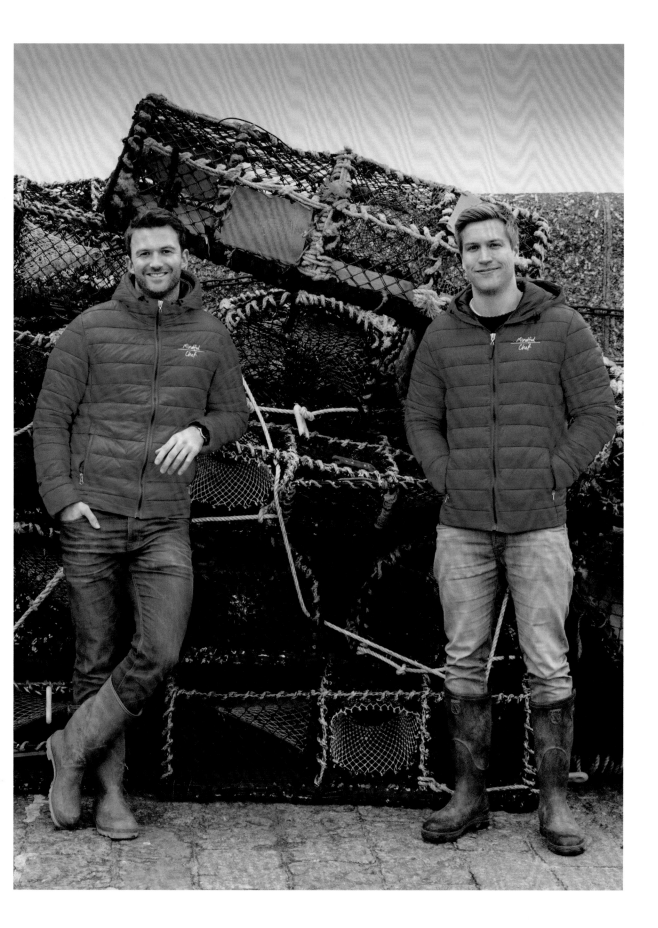

EATING THE MINDFUL CHEF WAY

WHAT SHOULD I EAT?

It has never been as easy to find information on healthy eating, however, the sheer amount posted online can often make what should be a relatively simple task seem like a daunting one, and you can struggle to find answers to some of the smallest questions. Following a specific diet or way of eating – whether it's Atkins, low-fat or Paleo – has always been popular in the UK, but today eating well and looking after our health has achieved an even bigger mainstream following, with a rising number of lifestyles and diets vying for our attention.

At Mindful Chef, we don't believe you should look at eating as a diet but as a way of fuelling your body. What you eat will determine how you look and feel. We include a range of proteins, carbohydrates and fats in all of our meals because to exclude one would limit the amount of vitamins and minerals the body receives. However, there is a difference between the types of proteins, carbohydrates and fats you can eat and this is where people often trip up.

• PROTEIN

Protein is essential if you want to live a long and healthy life. Protein helps your body recover from daily tasks and also helps the maintenance and growth of lean muscle. This becomes increasingly more important as we grow older as it is much harder to retain lean muscle mass and everyday life gets a little bit more difficult. Having more lean muscle will help support our joints and bones, both of which will also deteriorate as we age. Protein is made up of two types of amino acids – essential and non-essential amino acids – and these are the building blocks of muscle. Essential amino acids cannot be made by the body so we have to get them from our food. Animal protein is one of the easiest and most efficient ways of getting all the essential amino acids; with plant-based protein this is a bit more complex as not all sources contain all the essential amino acids. However, by eating and combining different sources of plant-based protein you are able to cover all of your bases and get the amino acids your body needs. The best plant-based sources of protein are a combination of pulses, beans, grains and tofu. Non-essential amino acids can be made by the body but it is best to try and support this process by including sources of in your diet – with foods such as nuts, grains, and a variety of fruit and vegetables.

• CARBOHYDRATES

If there is one food group that people stop eating immediately in a quick bid to lose weight it is more often than not carbohydrates. Most of the time they do see results and changes in their body composition, but these are only temporary. Carbohydrates help your body retain water so when you give them up completely you will end up looking somewhat thinner or firmer as your body retains less water. As you read on through this book though, you will begin to understand a bit more about the importance of carbohydrates in maintaining a healthy body. Carbohydrates are essential for good health and at Mindful Chef we like to put them into two groups – refined and unrefined. Refined carbohydrates are foods that have been altered in some way during the manufacturing process for human consumption.

Often refined carbohydrates are stripped of their nutrients and even have artificial flavourings and sugars added, which can cause havoc on our bodies by spiking sugar levels and are often the cause of many health problems. We make a point of not including foods like white bread, pies, pastries, battered foods or processed sauces high in refined carbohydrates in our meals for these very reasons, instead choosing to load our recipes with unrefined complex carbohydrates that are digested and absorbed by the body at a much slower pace, meaning they sustain our energy levels for longer. Our meals are therefore packed with whole grains such as millet, buckwheat and quinoa, as well as seasonal root vegetables like sweet potatoes and carrots, legumes, such as beans and lentils, and fruits.

• FATS

Fats are probably the most misunderstood food group of the three. Having been demonised by the media and government for decades, healthy fats are finally making a resurgence. With good reason too. If you want to be healthy then the right fats are going to play a major role in your diet. Conversely, when people eliminate fats from their diet they have to replace them with something else and usually it is foods riddled with 'hidden' sugar and refined carbohydrates. Not only is fat a great source of energy but it also forms our cells and in turn our brains and nervous systems. It is important to understand that there

are different types of fats and they perform different roles in the body. Unsaturated fats are the 'healthy' fats we need to be eating.

Monounsaturated fats can help reduce your levels of 'bad' cholesterol; avocados and olive oil are good examples. Cholesterol is very important for the body as it makes up a part of every cell membrane in the body and we can't function without it, so much so that our liver actually synthesises cholesterol itself everyday. Cholesterol is carried around the body in two forms – HDL (high density lipoprotein or 'good' cholesterol), which takes excess cholesterol back to the liver and gets rid of it; and LDL (low density lipoprotein or 'bad' cholesterol), which transports cholesterol from the liver to the rest of the body. Remember, cholesterol is important as it will help muscles grow and plays an important role in hormone function because it helps make up every cell of the body.

However, increased levels of 'bad' cholesterol in the body are a result of your body trying to fight problems such as inflammation. Inflammation occurs when your body reacts to foreign invaders like those found in trans-saturated fats (think crisps and chocolate). Cholesterol is sent to the arteries to heal inflammation but if you continue to fill your body with foreign invaders then inflammation will get worse and more cholesterol will be sent to try and stop it. This results in a build-up of cholesterol. If this happens, plaque can collect, clogging arteries and making them less flexible. In the worst cases this can lead to a clot forming, resulting in a heart attack or stroke. If there are no problems in the first place your body will not need to produce more cholesterol than it needs for daily functions and there won't be a build-up of 'bad' cholesterol.

Polyunsaturated fats can be found in foods containing omega-3 essential fatty acids (EFAs), such as salmon, mackerel, tuna, cod liver oil, walnuts, chia seeds and egg yolks. As their name suggests, these are vital for the body, yet we can't synthesise them ourselves. EFAs have been shown to help reduce the amount of inflammation in our body, as well as chronic diseases. Generally as a Western society our diets are very low in omega-3 fatty acids so it is a good idea to consciously make an effort to eat more foods containing them.

Saturated fats such as those found in butter, oil, red meat and coconut milk, have universally been regarded as unhealthy for some time now, with evidence that they can cause a higher rate of cardiovascular disease, diabetes and cancer. It is important to note that not all saturated fats are the same and many have actually been proven to lower the amount of 'bad' cholesterol in the body. Usually the argument against saturated fats is supported when there are other poor dietary choices, such as a diet high in refined carbohydrates, sugar and trans fats.

Trans fats are created through manufacturing, using a process called hydrogenation. Hydrogenation effectively changes the chemical configuration of a fat so it can harden at room temperature, therefore prolonging its shelf life. This means our bodies struggle to process them effectively, which can lead to a problems such as increased risk of heart disease and 'bad' cholesterol. Examples of trans fats are crisps, chocolate, battered foods and cakes.

- **WHOLE VS PROCESSED**

If there is one message we want you to take away from this book besides the fact that eating healthily eating can be easy, it would be this: replace processed foods with natural, whole foods. When we eat natural foods – fruit, vegetables, grains etc. – our hormones tell our brain when we are full and therefore that we should stop eating. Because processed foods have so many additives, preservatives and other chemicals they can actually suppress the hormones that tell the brain we are full. This often leads to overeating and consequently a higher risk of weight gain, insulin resistance and eventually obesity.

Processed foods are often much more calorific than natural foods but also a lot less nutritious. For example, a bag of sweets isn't going to offer much in terms of nutrition but they will be fairly high in the number of calories. They may give you a short burst of energy but they won't really satiate your hunger as the density or amount of food eaten is fairly small. Compare this to a salad of leafy greens and some good fats like olives or avocado. Both meals may contain a similar amount of calories but the second will help provide your body with all of the nutrients and vitamins it needs to perform at an efficient and optimal rate. The salad is also a greater volume of food, which will help you feel fuller as your body attempts to digest the food. You may have heard people say 'a calorie is a calorie' and it doesn't matter where you get it from as long as you don't overeat. This simply isn't the case. Sure coconut oil has a lot of calories and fat per gram but with each calorie comes a myriad of vitamins. So the next time you reach for a processed meal really think about what it might be doing to your body. Instead why not cook yourself a healthier version made from real, natural food.

OUR BELIEFS

When we started Mindful Chef it was with the intention of making healthy eating easy and in turn helping people to live better lives. Through our mission statement we believe that healthy eating will transcend into every aspect of people's lives, improving not only personal relationships but also how they cope with the stresses of everyday life. As you read on through this book you will start to understand more about the positive effects good nutrition can have on how you exercise, your sleep, productivity, stress levels and gut health.

- **GOOD FOR YOU, DELICIOUS AND QUICK**

Our recipes hold true to three core principles: they should be good for you, delicious and quick. Good for you means exactly that – foods that will help nurture your body and help its recovery. Foods that are natural, whole, unprocessed and provide you with all of vitamins and minerals you need to help your body function optimally.

Healthy eating doesn't have to bland or boring – it can actually taste delicious and be good for you. The fad diets and the idea that it's all chicken and broccoli is not the case. By gaining a few tips or knowing which spices and herbs to use with certain foods you can completely transform meals that you might think to be tasteless.

We know just how busy people's lives have become but we also know that so many time-poor people do have good intentions to try and eat healthily. This is why our recipes are all designed to be cooked in under 30 minutes from start to finish.

Aside from these three core beliefs, we want you to enjoy cooking. We think it should be a time to relax and disconnect from everything else that is going on in your life. Use it as a moment to lose yourself and enjoy the whole process; cooking doesn't have to be stressful or a chore. Everybody should be able to dedicate 30 minutes each night to cooking themselves a good, healthy meal – your body deserves it.

Finally, balance is key. When setting out on this journey Giles and I wanted to show people that living a healthier lifestyle can be a realistic and achievable goal, and for this we think balance is everything. Being your typical guys in their late twenties/early thirties we know that people are going to want to let their hair down every now and again and have an occasional beer or glass of wine. We also know that everyone is going to make some questionable food choices once in a while, or going to want to have some ice cream on a really hot day. Eating the Mindful Chef way isn't about punishing yourself or feeling like you've done something wrong. As long as we're eating well 80 per cent of the time we don't worry too much about the occasional pizza when out with friends. Life is to be enjoyed.

- **GLUTEN FREE AND DAIRY FREE**

All of our recipes are both gluten free and dairy free and we do this for a very specific reason. Food intolerances are rising as more and more people are increasingly aware of their body and how they feel. An intolerance can be something as small as feeling bloated, but it can also be as serious as coeliac disease – an autoimmune disease that damages the lining of the small intestine. Gluten and dairy have changed a lot in the last 100 years. Industrialisation and global demand have led to a dramatic change in farming methods and we believe that everyone can benefit from reducing the amount of gluten and dairy in their diets. By omitting these ingredients from our recipes we are able to cater for those who suffer from food intolerances so that everyone can cook delicious, healthy meals. Again it is all about balance – we know not everyone follows a gluten-free diet and a lot of people will use our recipes to eliminate these ingredients and eat healthily from Monday to Friday – but they might also eat a pizza or a burger at the weekend. We just think that by reducing the amount they eat they are less likely to develop any intolerances or feel the effects of them on a regular basis.

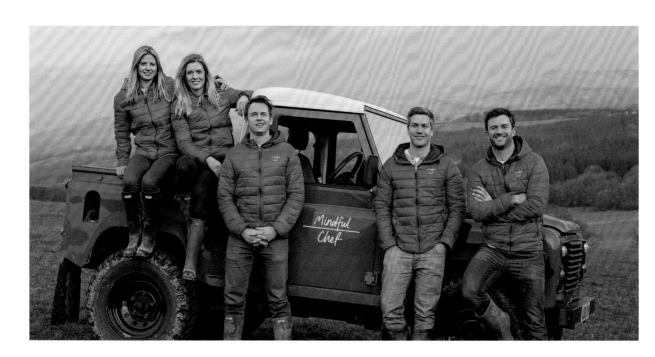

CALORIE COUNTING vs PORTION CONTROL

We aren't big calorie counters at Mindful Chef; instead we prefer to focus on portion sizes. There's so much confusion about the number of calories in food and the room for error is actually quite high. As such the numbers you may find in many apps or on the Internet might not be that accurate. Also far too many people get bogged down worrying over small numbers that in reality mean quite little. Remember a 'calorie isn't just a calorie'. Food quality and the amount of food you eat is far more important. When catering for so many people of different ages, sizes, genders and body shapes we find it is far better to look at portion sizes instead. This way you can be sure you are eating the same amount of food each time and you can adapt it to your personal requirements.

We like to use our hands as a measure of how much protein, carbohydrates and fat to eat at each meal. This is the following:

Women should eat 3–5 meals a day, using the guidelines below. Start with 3 meals a day. If however, you find you aren't eating enough or you are regularly exercising and need to eat more to help your body recover, increase this to 5 meals a day.

FOR WOMEN, EACH MEAL SHOULD CONSIST OF:

- 1 serving of protein – the size of your palm
- 1 serving of carbohydrates – the size of your cupped hand
- 1 serving of vegetables – the size of your fist
- 1 serving of fats – the size of your thumb

Men should eat 4–6 meals a day. They should start with 4 meals a day but again, this can be increased to 6 depending on how much you are exercising and what your goals are. Your meals should consist of:

FOR MEN, EACH MEAL SHOULD CONSIST OF:

- 1–2 servings of protein – the size of your palm
- 1–2 servings of carbohydrates – the size of your cupped hand
- 1–2 servings of vegetables – the size of your fist
- 1–2 servings of fats – the size of your thumb

How much you actually eat will depend on a variety of factors, including your goals, gender, body shape and body type. However, we think this eating plan can serve anyone well as a starting point. If you find you are putting on weight, either reduce the amount you eat by a meal or slightly reduce the portions you have at each meal. If you need to put on weight you can add a meal or increase your portion sizes. The best things about this are that anyone can do it; it's personalised and you don't need a phone or the Internet to track your calories.

It's really important to note that the above are merely guidelines – a starting point for you to work from if you wish. There is nothing scientifically groundbreaking in this book, nor are there any quick fixes. However, you will find a lot of advice on habitual changes that you can incorporate into your daily routine that may help improve the quality of your life. Your nutrition and health don't have to be complicated and feel like another task to add to your already busy schedule. They should be things that you want to make better and you should start to enjoy the process of feeling more energised, less stressed and, most importantly, healthier. We don't think you should have to give up anything – life is too short and we believe strongly in finding a balance. Eating healthily is something everyone can do and if you make a couple of small changes to how and what you eat, it can make a huge difference to your life.

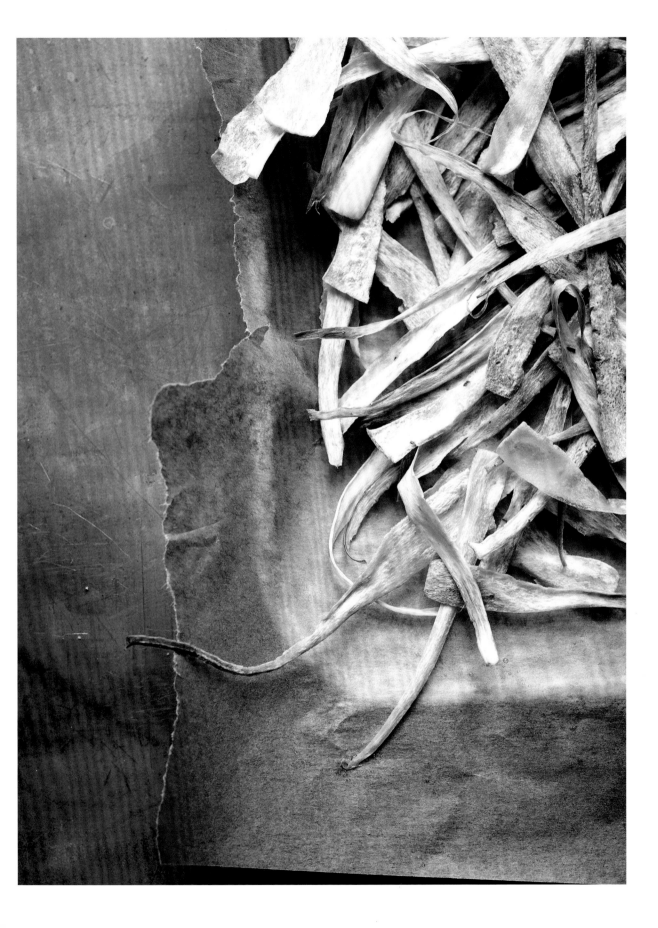

A MINDFUL WEEK

People often ask us what a week in the life of Myles and Giles looks like, so we thought we would put together an example of what we get up to in our day-to-day lives and how we approach a mindful week. The example below is what a typical week for Giles looks like, but really it's pretty similar for both of us.

The first thing to say is that it is incredibly difficult nowadays with all the distractions of modern technology and ever longer working hours to create a balanced lifestyle, but we passionately believe this is one of the fundamentals to a healthy happy life. We also know it is achievable; you just need a little planning.

• MONDAY

The week starts off with the delivery of a Mindful Chef box, loaded with fresh good-for-you ingredients and recipe cards. I like to go for four recipes a week as I'm usually busy towards the end of the week, seeing friends and being out and about. This keeps me on track Monday to Thursday, and means a regular healthy diet is achievable with little effort.

It is important to get the day off to the right start with a good breakfast, so I usually cycle to work and then have a bowl of oats and berries. Myles and I will then ensure that we hit the park for a workout at lunch, usually a HIIT session (high intensity interval training involving lots of bodyweight movement) or a run around the park. Some vitamin D and fresh air really clears the mind and helps focus on work in the afternoon.

In the evening it will be a cycle or run home and then a Mindful Chef box is in the fridge ready to be chopped, cooked and served up for dinner.

• TUESDAY

Once a month, towards the start of the week we get the office team to try a new workout, sport or exercise. There are so many innovative ways to stay fit and healthy these days that you really can learn a new activity every month. One that took me by surprise was Bikram yoga, which is yoga practised at 40°C. We'll start the day with one of these sessions at around 7am and then head to the office feeling fresh and ready to take on the day.

For lunch we will often be lucky enough to be tasting and testing new recipes created by our fabulous chef Louisa. Myles and I approve everything that goes into our dishes and we work closely with Louisa to bring the freshest and tastiest flavours to our recipes.

• WEDNESDAY

After working up an appetite by cycling to work I'll grab a quick scrambled eggs and leafy green vegetable breakfast. Some people say it is hard to eat well quickly in the morning. I disagree; if it isn't berries and oats, which is literally throwing something in a bowl, then why not try scrambled eggs with steamed veg? Five minutes and you have a nutritious breakfast which won't send your insulin levels through the roof and leave you craving naughty foods

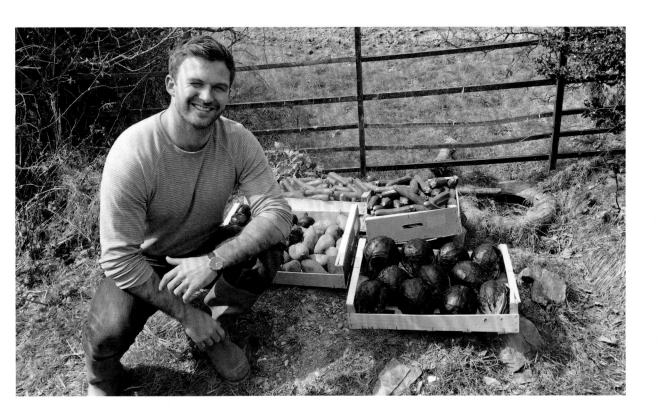

later. It's then off to the gym at lunch for an all-body conditioning session with Myles. We try to balance park workouts with the gym as it allows both indoor and outdoor exercise. Again this only needs to be an intense 30-minute session to get the heart rate going. I'll then grab a post-workout blueberry and banana smoothie which gets me through the day with a nice natural boost. Like with every other day in the week, sleep is hugely important (for more on this see chapter 5). Put simply, you have to allow your body to relax and recover fully otherwise you are not allowing it to prepare for the next day. Learn to turn off your phone, TV or other electronic device by a certain time – I like to aim for 10.30pm. Allow your mind to relax and unwind before you go to sleep. You'll notice huge changes in how you feel the next morning.

• THURSDAY

A study based on one million participants last year highlighted that we are not getting enough exercise per day and linked it to some pretty alarming statistics. The study recommended a minimum of one hour's exercise a day. We feel strongly about this and whether it is a cycle to work, a stroll around the park at lunch, or jogging home rather than using the car, it is important that people make time for this in their lives.

In the afternoon, to keep my body topped up after a jog around the park, I will tuck into a healthy snack, such as beef jerky, biltong or some nuts and seeds. There are some really tasty healthy snacks out there (see pages 204–214 for some of our recipes) so there really is no excuse to be constantly grabbing chocolate bars (except at Christmas!).
I also try and incorporate a little bit of stretching into my weekly routine, either pre-workout or at other down time; you'd be surprised what 5 minutes can do for your long-term health.

• FRIDAY

A spinach, tomato and mushroom omelette is my favourite way to kick-start Friday. If I'm feeling like treating myself then I'll add some smoked salmon for that extra boost of omega-3 fatty acids. Myles and I will often have meetings on Fridays (funny that people like to put in late-afternoon Friday meetings so that they can then slink off to the pub for a well-earned drink). We obviously enjoy a tipple now and again too – everything in moderation!

• SATURDAY

Usually from September to May I'm playing rugby, which means getting ready for a game in the morning with a full breakfast of oats followed by some scrambled eggs and bacon. If I'm not then I try to get out on the bike for a nice decent ride. Being a country boy in the city means I am constantly yearning for greenery and open space. London's parks may not quite look like the rolling hills of Devon but if you explore a little further you can find some absolutely beautiful cycle routes on which to put your foot to the pedal, so to speak. It's then about relaxing with mates, grabbing a drink and catching up on what is going on with the important things in life: friends and family.

• SUNDAY

This used to be an early rise for Myles and me as we would jump on our bikes and head down to the Mindful Chef operations centre to pack our customers' boxes ready for our fleet of couriers to pick them up and drop them all over the country. We don't personally do this every Sunday nowadays, so it is nice to enjoy a little down time. I'll usually wake and have a coffee (I'm a fan of a small company called Bean & Ground based in Devon near where I grew up) while reading the paper and enjoying a slower pace to the day. A walk around the local common and a catch up with more friends is always a nice way to while away a lazy Sunday afternoon. Then it's time for some 'life admin' in the evening, the usual sorting of yourself ready for the week ahead.

If there is one thing I've learnt, it is that a healthy life is about balance. Incorporate some of the above into your weekly routines and you'll really start to notice the difference.

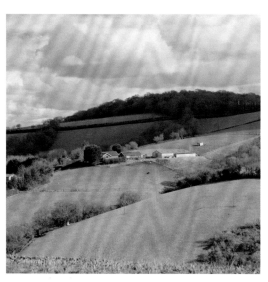

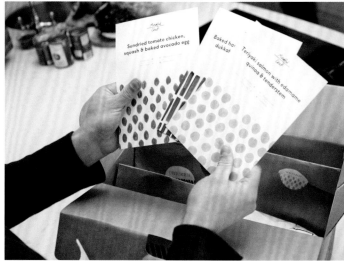

RECIPE NOTES

- All of our recipes are designed to be prepared and cooked quickly – within 30 minutes from start to finish.

- We advise using coconut oil or olive oil for their nutritional benefits. Coconut oil is naturally free from trans fatty acids and contains many health benefits once heated. It can help to control your blood sugar levels and provide you with energy. We cook with up to 1 tablespoon of oil per person per meal.

- We use sea salt because it contains many naturally occurring minerals and trace elements like potassium, calcium and magnesium. However, we advise keeping salt to a minimum, just use a pinch or two to bring out the flavours in the dish.

- Eggs are medium unless otherwise stated but it won't matt too much if you use a different size.

- When making vegetable noodles, it's handy to have a spiraliser, which will give you lovely, long uniform noodles, but a julienne peeler can also be used, or simply a Y-peeler, which will make wide ribbon-like noodles.

- Remember to wash all fruit and vegetables before preparing them, to remove any soil.

- The skins and peel of most vegetables are edible and contain many nutrients. Where possible leave these on when cooking, otherwise put them into your compost for making mineral-rich fertiliser.

- We try and keep washing-up to a minimum by using as little equipment as possible. However if you want to save time, you could blend the ingredients for some of the sauces like the pestos, and use a food processor for making cauliflower and broccoli rice instead of using a grater.

- We ensure all of our recipes are well balanced.

- All recipes serve 2 unless otherwise stated. They can be doubled or scaled up accordingly if you're serving more.

THE FIRST WEALTH
IS HEALTH

Ralph Waldo Emerson

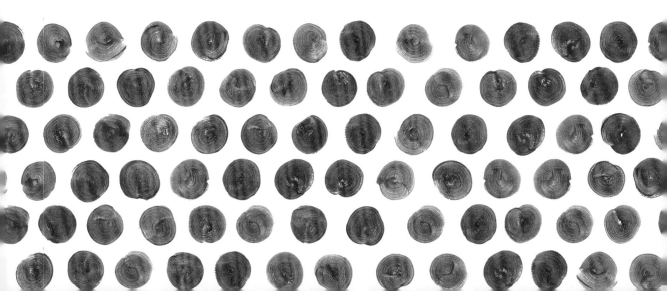

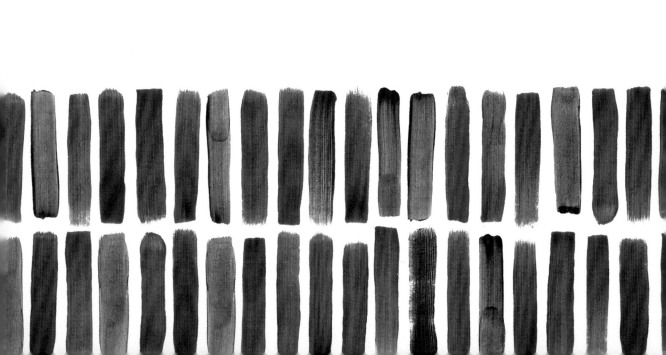

ENERGY
+
PRODUCTIVITY

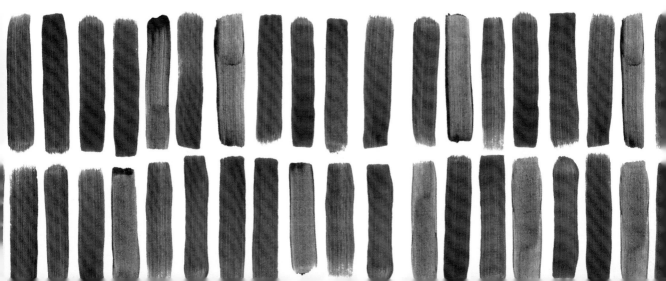

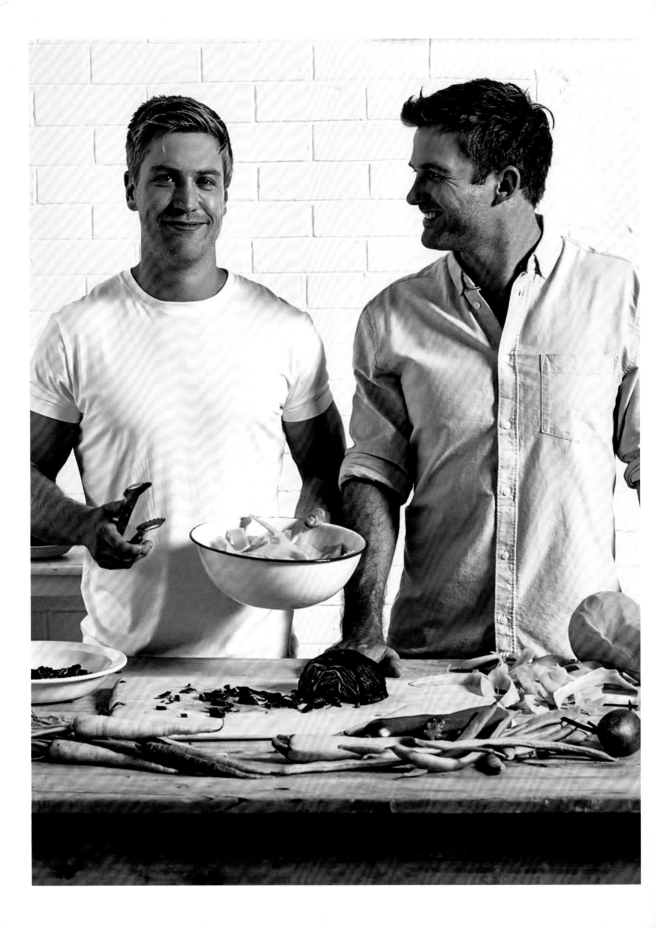

ENERGY + PRODUCTIVITY

People are working more and more hours in the day and this is having a direct impact on our health. Thanks to the internet and the development of smartphones, we are struggling to switch off properly. We're constantly thinking about work or the latest Instagram post we simply have to check. Our lives have become consumed by the virtual world, so it's no wonder we are struggling to find the time to disconnect and relax, let alone eat well and cook ourselves proper meals. One effect is that many of us feel our energy levels are flagging or we're simply not being that productive.

When we are busy, we stop thinking about what is most important to us and stop prioritising what our body needs to function at its best. Food is often the first element to be neglected, despite the fact that it is the thing that will enable us to power through stressful workloads and give us the energy we need to make ourselves more productive. After a long day at work, it is all too easy to grab an unhealthy, processed ready meal from the supermarket on the way home or to forget about eating entirely. We have all been guilty of this at one time or another (Giles and myself included), but working as a trainer and nutritional coach, I have experienced at first hand the benefits of regular, healthy eating and how it can transform people's lives for the better. If you can get into good habits, it will make such a difference to your energy levels and general well-being.

The main thing to consider is that food is fuel. You wouldn't fill up a Ferrari using sunflower oil instead of petrol, and our bodies respond in much the same way. Our bodies have a limited supply of energy and we rely on food to power us so that we can operate properly and perform the basic metabolic functions that keep our organs working the way they should. The types of food we eat play a huge role in determining how we are feeling (mentally and physically) and how we look; they affect our mood, our body weight and our hormonal status.

So how can nutrition make you a better, more energised, productive person and improve your quality of life on a daily basis?

FUELLING UP FOR THE DAY

In order for us to be more productive and improve our concentration levels, attention span and general mood, it is important to eat a good breakfast. Eating a healthy, balanced breakfast is your biggest weapon in getting your energy levels up and preparing your body to take on anything the day throws at you. The reason you hear so many people tell you that breakfast is the most important meal of the day is because it can affect your neurotransmitters – these are chemicals in the brain that send messages throughout your brain and body to help increase your attention span and concentration levels. Imagine going to work every day feeling alert and energised.

While an unhealthy breakfast – one that is poor in nutrient quality, such as sugary breakfast cereals (even the so called 'healthy' ones often contain lots of sugar!) – can leave you feeling tired, grumpy and send you on a blood-sugar rollercoaster, a healthy breakfast, such as the ones I've suggested opposite, full of protein, slow-release carbohydrates and good fats, allows a slow and steady rise in blood sugar. As their name implies, this type of carbohydrate releases energy to your body slowly, meaning you have a steady supply of energy for longer and

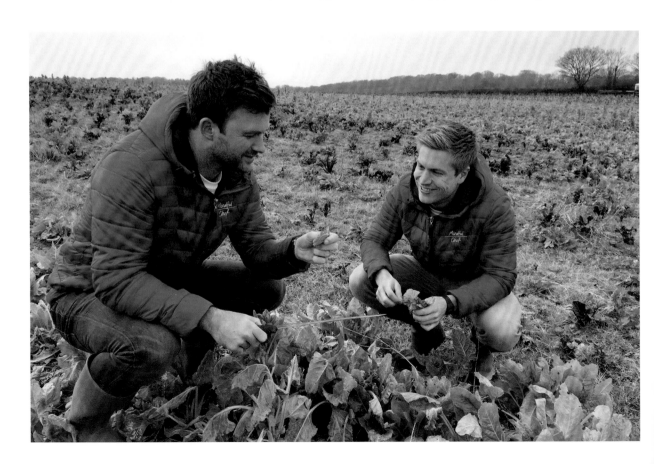

won't be reaching for a quick boost, such as a chocolate bar, an hour after you've eaten. The healthy fats, such as monounsaturated fats, found in avocados, help slow the release of sugars into the bloodstream, prompting less insulin release.

HERE ARE SOME OF MY FAVOURITE HEALTHY BREAKFASTS:

- Crunchy pecan, coconut & chia granola (see page 46)
- Mexican veggie breakfast (see page 50)
- Sweet potato & ginger röstis with crushed avocado and tenderstem (see page 52)

KEEPING ENERGISED

Energy in comes from the food you eat and energy out will be determined by the body's needs to function, exercise, digest food and survive. You can enter two states of energy balance – negative or positive. Negative energy balance is a result of not eating enough calories for your daily needs, and a positive energy balance occurs when you overeat. Being in either can affect your body's functions (your metabolism, for example), and a skewed energy balance can affect our mood too. Take a negative energy balance: to lose weight lots of people will focus solely on eating less food without taking into account the types of food they're eating or other factors that could help them lose weight instead, such as exercising more regularly. By eating less than your daily needs you will lose weight, but you will also experience mood swings, a decline in metabolism and decreased hormone function. If you aren't eating enough calories for your body's needs the body will start to shut down non-critical functions, hence the decline in things like your thyroid hormones and metabolism. If weight loss is your goal, you are far better off creating a negative energy balance by exercising more while still eating enough calories to maintain your body's usual daily needs without having to shut down non-critical functions. The simplest way to explain this is that you will have to take note of how you look and feel to determine the amount of calories you really need on a daily basis. If your goal is to lose weight and you are putting on weight, you need to eat less. However, if you're losing weight but experiencing mood swings, if you're more tired than usual or are finding your weight loss is starting to plateau, it may be because you aren't actually eating enough to allow your body to perform all the daily processes it needs to. There is a lot of trial and error to find what really works for you and your body.

ENERGY AND APPETITE

Good nutrition throughout the day is essential for providing energy and controlling our appetites. Food that keeps us full should be high in fibre, vitamins and minerals; it should also have volume, as it is nutrient density and volume that keeps us full rather than calories. Take a chocolate bar, fizzy drink and a bag of crisps versus a huge bowl of salad with a healthy balance of protein, carbohydrates and fats (or a meal like the one of the lunches opposite). While both will likely have similar amounts of calories, one meal will leave you feeling full while the other offers very little nutritional value whatsoever, or volume in return for the amount of calories ingested, and you will most likely feel hungry again in an hour.

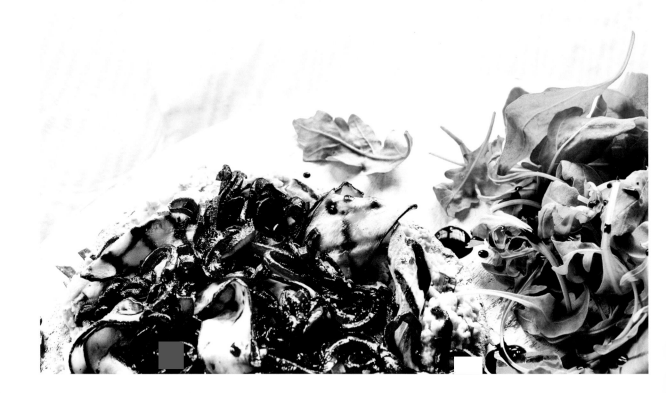

By focusing on thinking about the nutritional quality of food, rather than counting calories, you'll provide your body with the nutrients it needs to function optimally, you can ensure you eat the right amount of food for your energy needs, your productivity and energy levels will increase and you'll feel fuller for longer.

WINDING DOWN

Not only is food important for regulating your energy levels throughout the day, it also helps set your body up for sleep. If you have provided your body with the right nutrition during the day you will be helping it perform all of the functions it needs to while you are sleeping: functions such as aiding recovery, regulating hormone production and helping to restore bones and organs. In chapter 5, dedicated to sleep, I discuss exactly how food and sleep can make you healthier and that chapter contains a whole range of meals I like to eat before going to bed. They give me the vitamins and minerals I need to ensure I get a good night's sleep and that my body is able to recover and refuel properly before the morning.

TOP TIPS FOR MAINTAINING ENERGY AND PRODUCTIVITY THROUGHOUT YOUR DAY

1. **FOCUS ON INGREDIENTS, NOT COUNTING CALORIES**
   Calories are not solely to blame for skewed energy balance; it is a combination of the food we eat and the lifestyles we lead.

2. **PREPARATION IS KEY. FAIL TO PREPARE – PREPARE TO FAIL**
   I am lucky to be able to enjoy quality, nutritious food every day. However, before Mindful Chef I would make my own food and I still believe this is the most important rule you can follow for optimal health.

3. **EAT NUTRITIOUS FOOD THAT WILL ALLOW YOU TO EAT MORE AND SATIATE YOUR HUNGER**
   By doing this you won't find yourself reaching for unhealthy quick fixes like crisps and chocolate bars. They may give you a sudden increase of energy but they won't satisfy your hunger and you are likely to overeat.

All the meals included in this chapter have been designed to keep your energy and productivity at a stable and constant level. By including nutritious ingredients, these recipes will help satiate your hunger and you won't experience the blood-sugar rollercoaster you find with most processed foods.

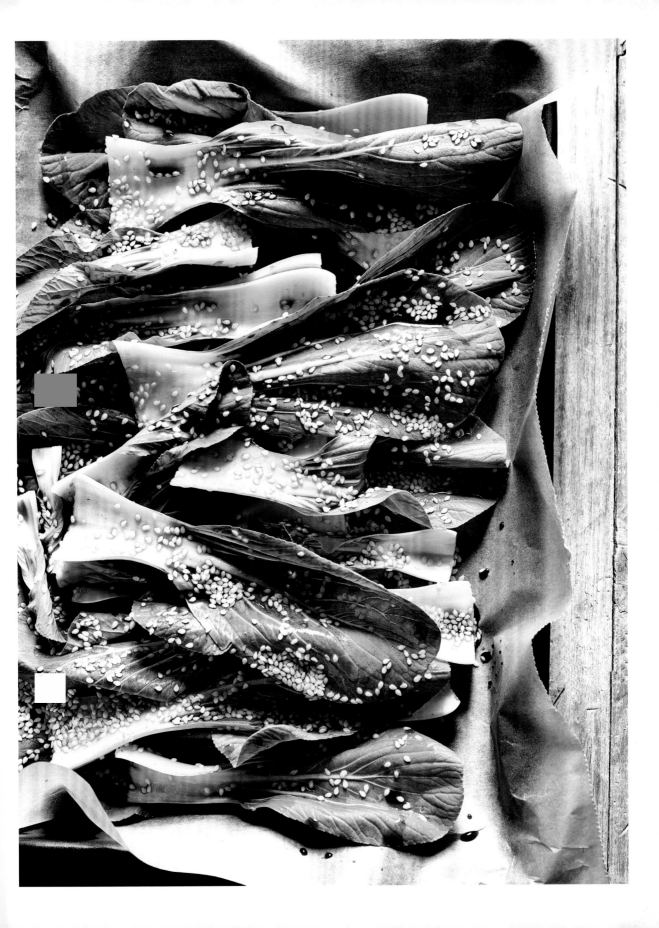

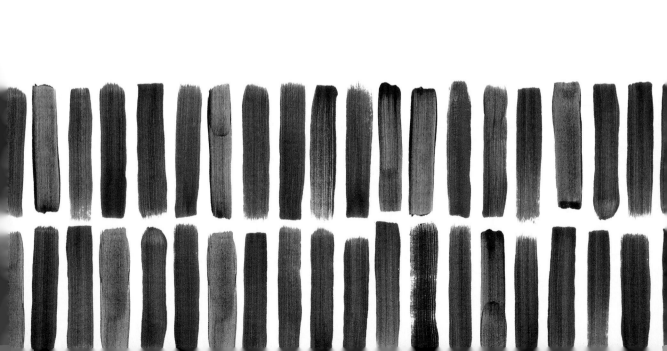

PEOPLE WHO LOVE TO EAT ARE ALWAYS THE BEST PEOPLE

Julia Child

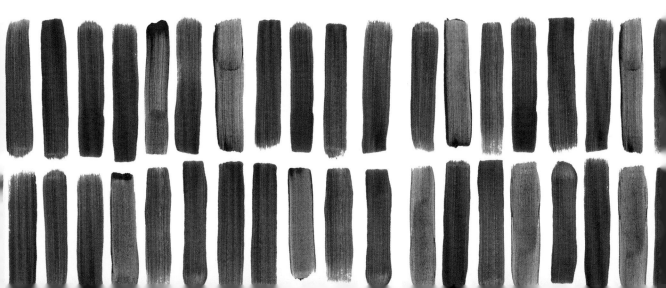

Chia seeds have become one of the most popular superfoods, as they are packed with fibre, protein, vitamins and omega-3 fatty acids, and are an excellent source of energy. The great thing about making homemade granola is that you can add any nuts or seeds you have left over in your kitchen. Be wary of buying shop-bought granola, as it's usually loaded with sugar. We top our granola with a big spoonful of thick and creamy coconut yoghurt, fresh berries for antioxidants and a sprinkle of cinnamon for speeding up the metabolism, setting us up well for the day ahead.

CRUNCHY PECAN, COCONUT & CHIA GRANOLA

100g gluten-free oats
70g pecans
30g flaked almonds
20g sunflower seeds
20g pumpkin seeds
20g chia seeds
20g desiccated coconut
2 tsp ground cinnamon
pinch of sea salt
1½ tbsp maple syrup
2 tbsp coconut oil (in liquid form
    – you may have to heat it
    gently until it turns liquid)
20g raisins

1 Preheat the oven to 180°C/gas mark 4.

2 Place the oats, pecans, flaked almonds, seeds, desiccated coconut, cinnamon and salt in a bowl and stir to combine.

3 In a separate bowl, mix together the maple syrup and coconut oil. Pour this into the dry ingredients and stir until fully combined.

4 Place the mixture on a sheet of baking paper on a baking tray. Spread the granola mixture out evenly and bake for 20 minutes, giving the mixture a shake halfway through.

5 Allow the granola to cool before stirring in the raisins and storing in an airtight container.

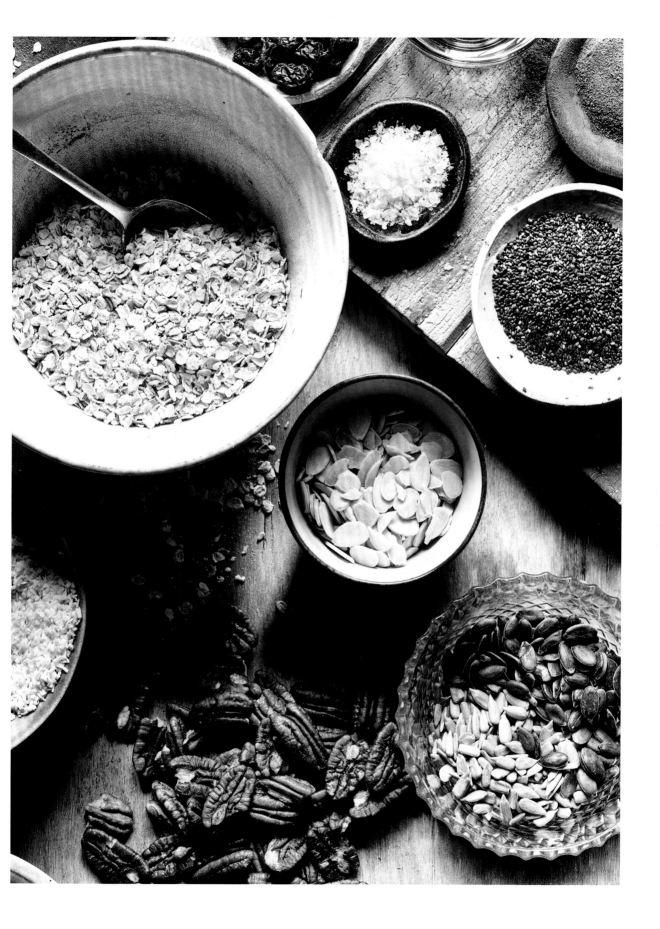

These pancakes are not only a brunch and breakfast favourite, but make a delicious dessert too, keeping you full for hours afterwards thanks to the protein-packed ingredients. They are super-speedy and can be made in just 15 minutes! This recipe makes 4 pancakes, 2 per person, and they are delicious drizzled with a little maple syrup, a natural sugar containing antioxidants.

BLUEBERRY & BANANA PROTEIN PANCAKES

2 ripe bananas
2 eggs
2 tbsp ground flaxseeds
2 tbsp ground almonds
handful of blueberries
coconut oil
2 tbsp maple syrup (optional)

1 Peel the bananas and mash in a bowl.

2 In a separate bowl, whisk the eggs with a fork.

3 To make the pancake batter, mix the eggs into the mashed banana and add the ground flaxseeds and ground almonds. Stir in the blueberries.

4 Heat a frying pan on a medium heat with ½ tablespoon of oil (you'll need to cook them in batches) and spoon in a quarter of the mixture for each pancake. Cook for 2–3 minutes each side, until turning golden brown.

5 Serve the pancakes as they are, or drizzled with the maple syrup.

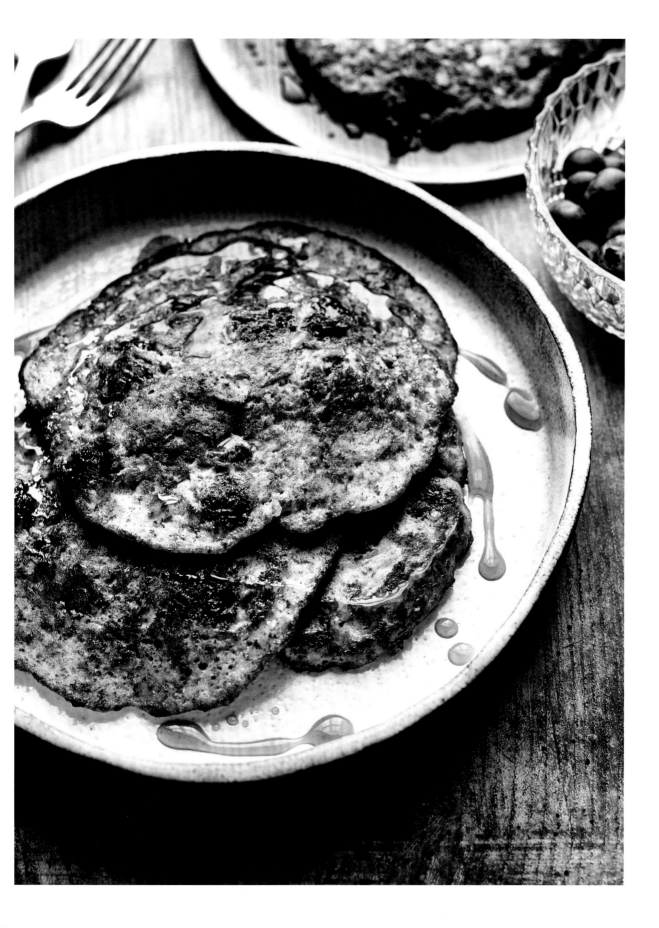

A nourishing, super-tasty and well-balanced vegetarian breakfast, full of good fats, iron and protein. Smoky fibre-rich black beans are spiced with paprika and chilli flakes to fire up your metabolism, and mixed with wilted spinach. We've topped the black beans with sliced avocado, fresh tomato salsa and soft poached eggs.

MEXICAN VEGGIE BREAKFAST

2 spring onions
120g ripe plum tomatoes
handful of fresh coriander
juice of 1 lime
coconut oil
240g drained black beans
½ tsp smoked paprika
¼ tsp chilli flakes
80g spinach
2 eggs
1 avocado
sea salt and black pepper

1 To make the tomato salsa, finely slice the spring onions, dice the tomatoes and roughly chop the coriander, then place in a bowl with half the lime juice.

2 Heat 1 teaspoon of oil in a frying pan on a low–medium heat. Add the drained black beans, smoked paprika and chilli flakes, season with sea salt and black pepper and cook for 5 minutes. Add the spinach and cook for a further 2 minutes, until wilted. Stir in the remaining lime juice.

3 Meanwhile bring a saucepan of water to a gentle simmer. Create a gentle whirlpool in the pan with a spoon, then carefully break the eggs into the middle, one at a time. Cook for 3–4 minutes, until the white is cooked, then remove from the pan.

4 Peel and de-stone the avocado and thinly slice.

5 Place the spicy black beans on warm plates, layer over the avocado slices, spoon over the fresh tomato salsa and top with the poached eggs.

6 Sprinkle with a pinch of sea salt and black pepper and serve.

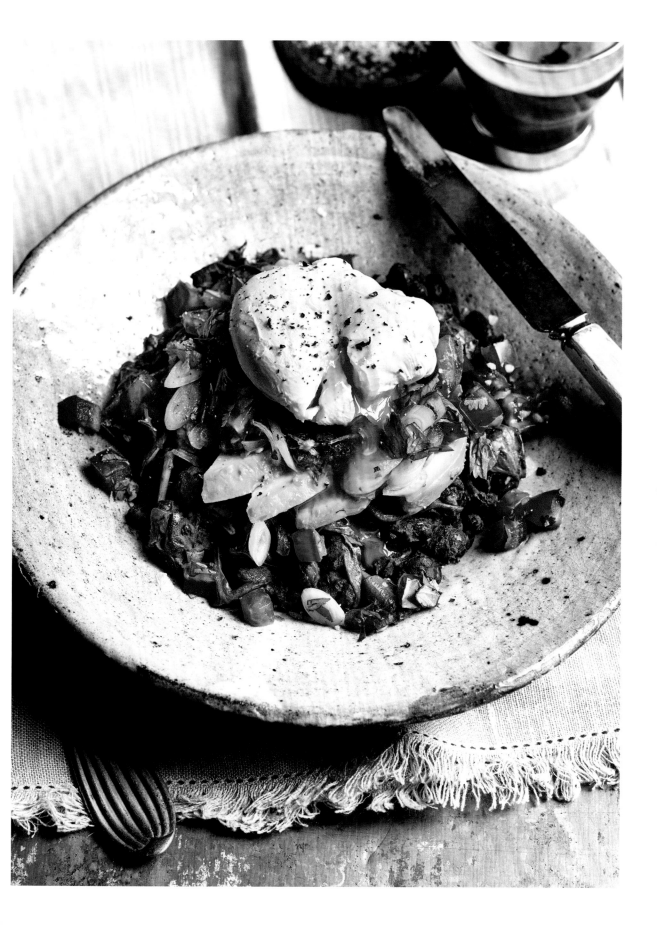

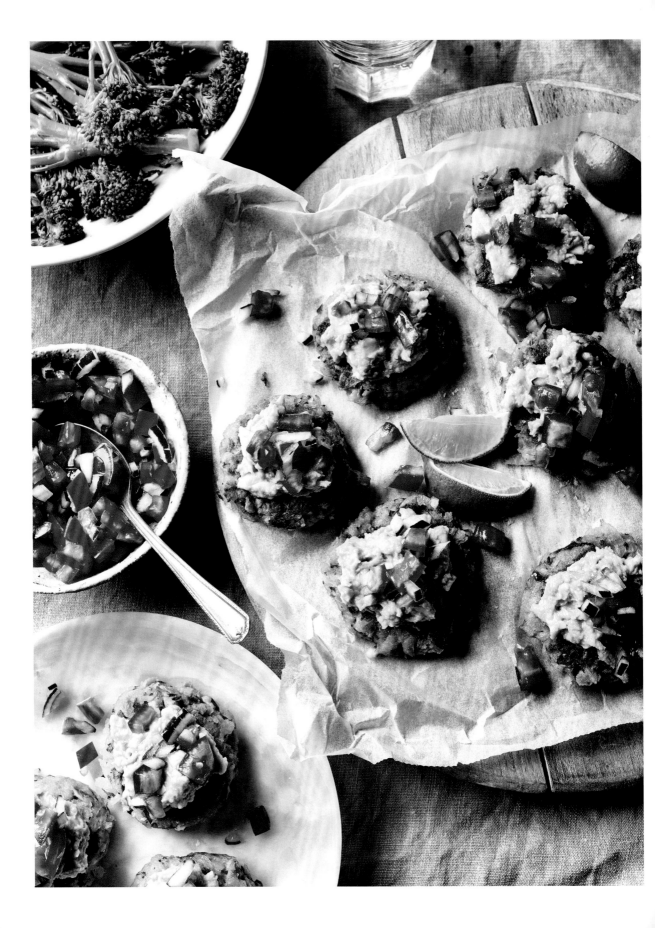

This is an incredibly tasty brunch but it's so satisfying it can be enjoyed at lunch or dinner too. The zingy fresh ginger and heat of the chilli works beautifully well with the creamy crushed avocado and a refreshing ripe tomato and red onion salsa. If you're looking for a protein hit, top the röstis with two oozing poached eggs, it will taste amazing and will set you up for the rest of the day.

SWEET POTATO & GINGER RÖSTIS WITH CRUSHED AVOCADO & TENDERSTEM

300g sweet potatoes
1 red onion
4cm fresh ginger
½ fresh red chilli
handful of fresh coriander
coconut oil
4 tbsp chickpea flour
200g tenderstem broccoli
1 avocado
2 tomatoes
juice of 1 lime, plus extra wedges
    to serve
sea salt and black pepper

1 Peel and grate the sweet potatoes and dice the red onion. Peel and finely chop the ginger and finely chop the red chilli and coriander.

2 Heat 1 teaspoon of oil in a large frying pan on a medium heat and fry the ginger, chilli, grated sweet potato and half the red onion for 5 minutes, until softened.

3 Transfer the contents of the pan to a bowl, add the coriander and chickpea flour, mix well and season. Form into 6 round shapes 1cm thick.

4 Heat 1 tablespoon of oil in the same frying pan on a medium-high heat and fry the röstis for 3–4 minutes each side, until golden brown.

5 Meanwhile, trim the tenderstem broccoli. Place in a steamer over a saucepan of boiling water, cover and cook for 5–7 minutes until cooked, then set aside and keep warm.

6 Peel and de-stone the avocado and crush it in a bowl with a fork, then season with salt and pepper. To make the salsa, finely chop the tomatoes and in a separate bowl mix them with the remaining red onion and half the lime juice.

7 To serve, top each rösti with a spoonful of crushed avocado and a spoonful of salsa and drizzle over the rest of the lime juice. Serve the tenderstem and remaining salsa alongside.

We prefer to use plant-based carbs rather than heavy pasta, which is why you'll find a range of our favourite 'spiralised' courgette and carrot dishes throughout the book. For our lasagne we favour the aubergine – deep purple in colour and packed with antioxidants to help balance blood sugar levels. We bake slices of aubergine to act as lasagne sheets and then layer these between a rich tomato and cannellini bean ragù and a chunky homemade basil and pine nut pesto. Meat-eaters will love this satisfying lasagne, which looks impressive and is one of our dinner party favourites.

VEGGIE LASAGNE WITH AUBERGINE, CANNELLINI BEAN RAGÙ & PESTO

2 garlic cloves
1 red onion
150g carrots
2 aubergines
olive oil
240g drained cannellini beans
200g tomato passata
2 tbsp balsamic vinegar
handful of fresh basil
30g pine nuts
handful of rocket
sea salt and black pepper

1 Preheat the oven to 200°C/gas mark 6.

2 Finely chop the garlic and finely dice the red onion and carrots. To make the aubergine lasagne layers, thinly slice the aubergines lengthways (you need at least 6 slices from each one).

3 Heat 1 teaspoon of oil in a medium-sized pan and fry the red onion and garlic for 3 minutes, then add the carrot and cook for 5 minutes.

4 Meanwhile, place 12 aubergine slices on a baking tray and drizzle with 2 teaspoons of oil and a pinch of sea salt. Cook in the oven for 10–15 minutes, turning the slices halfway through.

5 Add the cannellini beans to the pan of onion and carrot, along with the passata and a third of the balsamic vinegar. Season and simmer for 10 minutes.

6 Meanwhile, for the pesto, finely chop the basil and half the pine nuts, mix with 1 tablespoon of olive oil and season with salt and pepper.

7 When the aubergine slices are cooked, construct each lasagne by placing two pieces of aubergine parallel on the plate as the base. Add a generous spoonful of the bean sauce and a thin layer of pesto, and repeat. Top each lasagne with a final layer of aubergine slices. Sprinkle the rocket with the remaining pine nuts and balsamic vinegar.

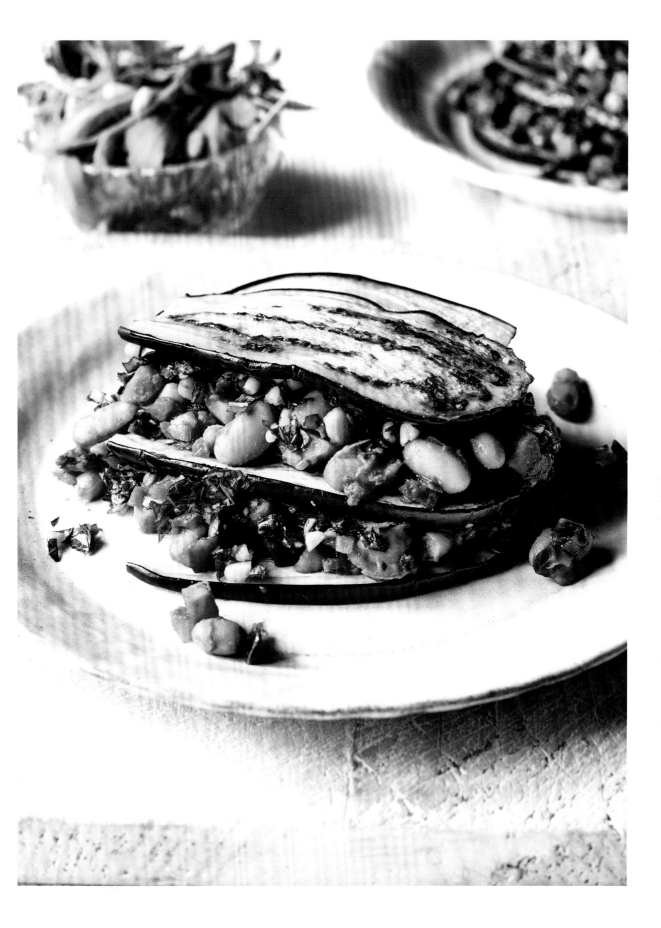

Californian cuisine is usually light and healthy, and a fusion of different styles. The umami-rich sweet miso paste and fresh chilli make a rich spicy dressing for the buckwheat noodles, vibrant veggies and sautéd tofu. Buckwheat noodles are a tasty gluten-free alternative to wheat noodles. They do have a tendency to stick together, so it's worth stirring them occasionally in the first few minutes of cooking and making sure they are rinsed in cold water afterwards.

CALIFORNIAN-STYLE BUCKWHEAT NOODLES WITH TOFU, CARROT & MISO DRESSING

300g firm tofu
150g carrots
1 fresh red chilli
200g courgettes
coconut oil
1 tbsp tamari
120g buckwheat noodles
2 tbsp sweet miso paste
2 tsp maple syrup
juice of 1 lime
handful of fresh mint
sea salt

1 Drain and rinse the tofu, then pat dry with kitchen paper. Cut into pieces about 1cm thick.

2 Peel the carrots and cut into matchsticks. Finely chop the chilli (remove the seeds for less heat). Remove the ends of the courgettes, but leave the skin on. Prepare courgette ribbons using a peeler.

3 Heat 1 tablespoon of oil in a frying pan on a medium heat and fry the tofu for 5 minutes. Add the tamari and fry for a further 2 minutes, then add the carrot matchsticks and fry for another 3 minutes, until the carrot has softened slightly.

4 Bring a pan of water to the boil and add the buckwheat noodles with a pinch of sea salt. Stir, then simmer for 5 minutes. Once cooked, rinse briefly in cold water and set aside.

5 Meanwhile, to make the sauce, mix the miso paste with the maple syrup and lime juice.

6 In a bowl, mix the noodles with the tofu, carrots, courgette ribbons and chopped chilli. Roughly tear the mint leaves, add to the bowl with the miso sauce and stir to combine. Serve on warm plates.

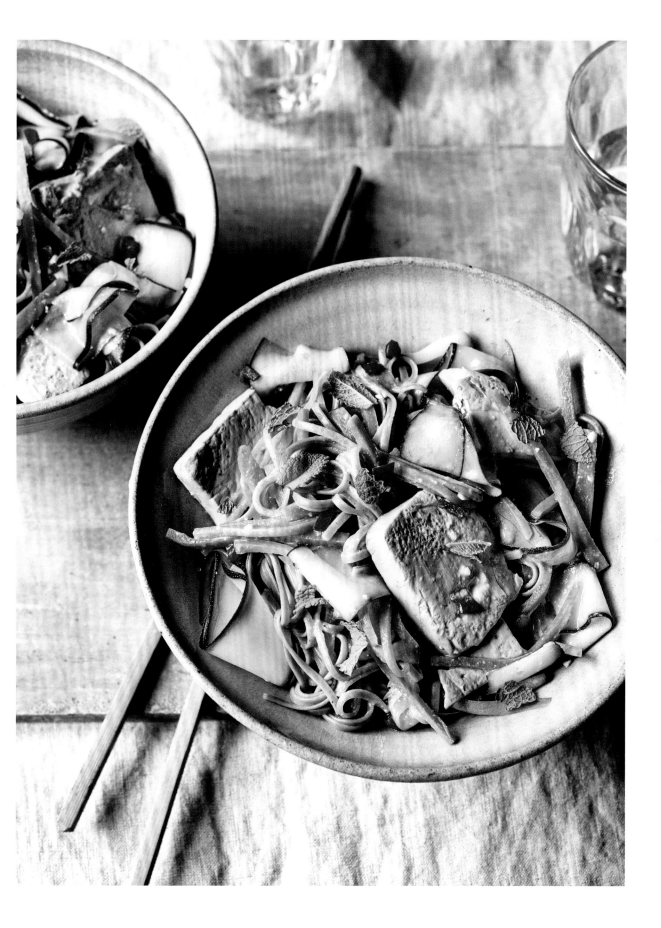

Fennel has many health benefits, including high levels of potassium for relaxing blood vessels, which in turn reduces blood pressure. Coupled with the beetroot in the falafels, which contains a large amount of folic acid for creating and maintaining cells, this is a super-healthy meal that will leave you feeling revitalised.

BEETROOT FALAFELS ON PARSLEY QUINOA WITH FENNEL & ORANGE SLAW

80g quinoa
300ml boiling water
2 garlic cloves
a handful of fresh flat-leaf parsley
240g drained chickpeas
200g beetroot
2 tbsp chickpea flour
2 tsp cumin seeds
2 tbsp tahini
olive oil
1 head of fennel
1 orange
sea salt and black pepper

1 Preheat the oven to 200°C/gas mark 6.

2 Rinse the quinoa, then place in a pan with the boiling water and simmer for 15 minutes until cooked. Meanwhile, crush or finely chop the garlic and finely chop the parsley.

3 Place the drained chickpeas in a bowl, then mash for a minute with a potato masher or the back of a fork until they are all crushed. Peel and grate the beetroot and add to the bowl.

4 Add the chickpea flour, garlic, cumin seeds, half the tahini and half the chopped parsley. Add ½ tablespoon of olive oil, season with sea salt and black pepper and mix well.

5 Form the chickpea mixture into 12 balls and place on a baking tray. Bake in the oven for 15–20 minutes, turning halfway through.

6 Meanwhile, very finely slice the fennel. Peel the orange and slice into segments. Mix the fennel and orange together in a bowl with the remaining tahini, ½ tablespoon of olive oil and a pinch of sea salt.

7 Drain the cooked quinoa, season with salt and pepper, and stir in the remaining parsley. Spoon the parsley quinoa on to a warm plate, and top with the beetroot falafels alongside the fennel and orange slaw.

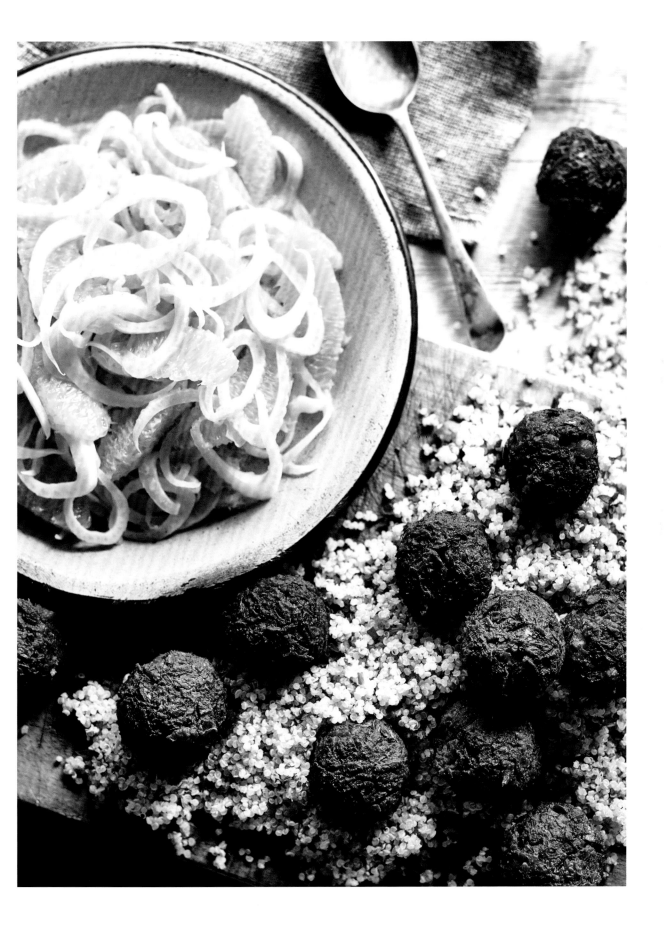

Our creamy veggie Malaysian laksa is the ultimate fresh and healthy comfort food. Infused with lemongrass, ginger and tamarind paste, we replace the more traditional wheat or rice noodles with mineral-dense carrots for an extra dose of nutrients, especially beneficial to vision. The warming soup will awaken your senses and make you feel energised.

MALAYSIAN TOFU & CARROT NOODLE LAKSA WITH FLAKED ALMONDS

1 fresh lemongrass stalk
4cm fresh ginger
2 garlic cloves
1 fresh red chilli
100g tenderstem broccoli
300g carrots
300g firm tofu
coconut oil
1 vegetable stock cube
200ml boiling water
200ml coconut milk
½ tsp tamarind paste
10g flaked almonds
sea salt and black pepper

1 Trim the ends of the lemongrass, remove the outer layer and finely chop. Peel and finely chop the ginger and garlic and finely slice the chilli (remove the seeds for less heat). Trim the ends of the tenderstem broccoli and cut in half.

2 Peel the carrots and trim the root ends. Prepare the carrot noodles by peeling them into ribbons, then slicing these lengthways into thin strips (or use a julienne peeler or spiraliser if you have one). Drain and rinse the tofu, then cut into 2cm cubes. Pat dry with kitchen paper.

3 Heat ½ tablespoon of oil in a frying pan on a medium heat and fry the tofu for 10 minutes, turning occasionally. Season with salt and pepper.

4 Dissolve the stock cube in the boiling water.

5 Heat 1 teaspoon of oil in a medium-sized pan. Add the lemongrass, ginger and garlic and fry for 2 minutes, then add the tenderstem and fry for a further 3 minutes. Add the coconut milk, vegetable stock, tamarind paste and carrot noodles. Bring to a simmer and cook for 5 minutes, then stir in the tofu.

6 Spoon the laksa into warm bowls and scatter over the flaked almonds and the sliced red chilli.

This Moroccan-spiced hearty fish stew is packed full of fibre-rich chickpeas, which provide a satisfying texture and nutty flavour along with a dose of vitamin E to help protect the heart. We've opted for monkfish tail, which provides useful vitamins needed for healthy brain function, and chunks of sweet roasted squash, simmered in a spicy tomato sauce with a sprinkling of flat-leaf parsley for added flavour.

MOROCCAN CHICKPEA & MONKFISH STEW WITH ROASTED SQUASH

2 garlic cloves
1 red onion
240g cherry tomatoes
handful of fresh flat-leaf parsley
300g monkfish
300g butternut squash
olive oil
1 tsp ras el hanout
1 vegetable stock cube
200ml boiling water
240g drained chickpeas
80g spinach
sea salt and black pepper

1 Preheat the oven to 180°C/gas mark 4.

2 Finely chop the garlic and thinly slice the red onion. Cut the cherry tomatoes in half and roughly chop the parsley. Slice the monkfish into bite-sized pieces.

3 Peel the squash and cut into 1cm cubes. Place on a baking tray and toss with 1 teaspoon of oil and a sprinkle of sea salt. Place in the oven for 15–20 minutes, turning halfway through cooking.

4 Meanwhile, heat 1 teaspoon of oil in a large pan on a medium heat. Add the garlic and red onion and cook for 5 minutes until softened. Stir in the ras el hanout and cherry tomatoes and cook for a further 2 minutes.

5 Meanwhile, dissolve the vegetable stock in the boiling water.

6 Add the drained chickpeas, vegetable stock and spinach to the pan of vegetables and cook for 5 minutes, until the sauce has reduced slightly.

7 Season the monkfish pieces with sea salt and black pepper and add to the pan, stirring the monkfish into the sauce. Place a lid on the pan and simmer for 8–10 minutes, until the fish is cooked through. Stir in the roasted squash and half the parsley.

8 Spoon the stew into warm bowls and scatter over the remaining parsley.

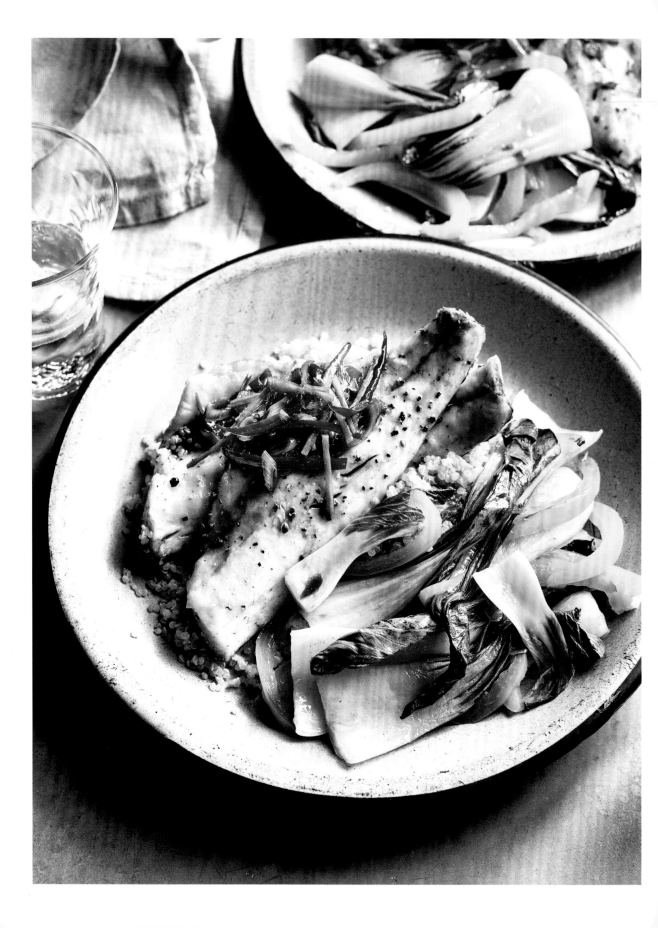

In this recipe we've paired lightly pan-fried sea bass with warm and fragrant ginger and sliced spring onion. Spring onions, like the rest of the onion family, contain powerful sulphur compounds, which have impressive antibacterial and antiviral properties for helping to ward off illnesses. The sweet miso and lime-infused quinoa has an addictive richness that pairs perfectly with refreshing pak choi.

GINGER & SPRING ONION SEA BASS WITH MISO & LIME QUINOA

80g quinoa
300ml boiling water
1 head of pak choi
1 yellow pepper
4cm fresh ginger
4 spring onions
½ fresh red chilli
coconut oil
2 x 150g sea bass fillets
2 tsp tamari
1 tbsp sweet miso paste
juice of ½ lime
sea salt and black pepper

1 Rinse the quinoa and put into a saucepan with the boiling water. Simmer for 15–20 minutes, until cooked.

2 Meanwhile, cut the root end off the pak choi and thinly slice the yellow pepper. Peel the ginger and slice into thin matchsticks. Finely slice the spring onions and red chilli lengthways.

3 Heat ½ tablespoon of oil in a frying pan on a medium heat. Add the pak choi and yellow pepper and cook for 5 minutes, until softened, then remove from the pan and keep warm.

4 Season the sea bass with sea salt and black pepper. Using the same frying pan, heat ½ tablespoon of oil on a medium heat and place the sea bass in the pan skin side down. Fry for 2–3 minutes each side, until cooked through. Remove from the pan.

5 Add 1 teaspoon of oil to the frying pan on a medium-high heat and add the ginger, chilli, spring onion and tamari. Cook for 3 minutes, until golden brown.

6 When the quinoa is cooked, drain, season and stir in the miso paste and lime juice.

7 To serve, place the miso and lime quinoa on a plate, top with the sea bass and spoon over the spring onions, chilli and ginger. Serve alongside the stir-fried pak choi and yellow pepper.

Sweet miso paste is a popular Japanese seasoning made from fermented soybeans – it makes a delicious partner to fish but also tastes incredible when smothered on roasted aubergine. For this dish, we've made a quick pickle of sliced cucumber and bright red radishes with white wine vinegar, which cuts through the sweet-salty richness of the miso beautifully.

SWEET MISO HAKE WITH PAK CHOI, PICKLED CUCUMBER & BLACK RICE

100g black rice
400ml boiling water
2 tbsp white wine vinegar
2 tsp honey
1 baby cucumber
100g radishes
1 head of pak choi
2 x 150g hake fillets
2 tbsp sweet miso paste
1 tbsp tamari
coconut oil
10g white sesame seeds
sea salt and black pepper

1 Preheat the oven to 180°C/gas mark 4.

2 Rinse the rice, put it into a saucepan with the boiling water and a pinch of salt, then simmer for 25–30 minutes, until the rice is cooked.

3 To make the pickled cucumber and radish, mix the white wine vinegar and honey in a bowl. Thinly slice the cucumber and radishes (removing any green stalks). Place the sliced cucumber and radishes in the bowl with the honey and vinegar, stir to coat and season with salt and pepper. Leave to pickle until needed.

4 Slice the end off the pak choi and separate the leaves.

5 Coat the top of each hake fillet with 1 tablespoon of sweet miso paste and place on a baking tray lined with baking paper. Bake in the oven for 15 minutes, until the fish is cooked through. At the same time, put the pak choi on a second baking tray, drizzle over the tamari, 1 tablespoon of oil and the sesame seeds, and bake for 15 minutes.

6 Drain the black rice.

7 To serve, place the pak choi on a warm plate and top with the hake. Serve the black rice and pickled cucumber and radish alongside.

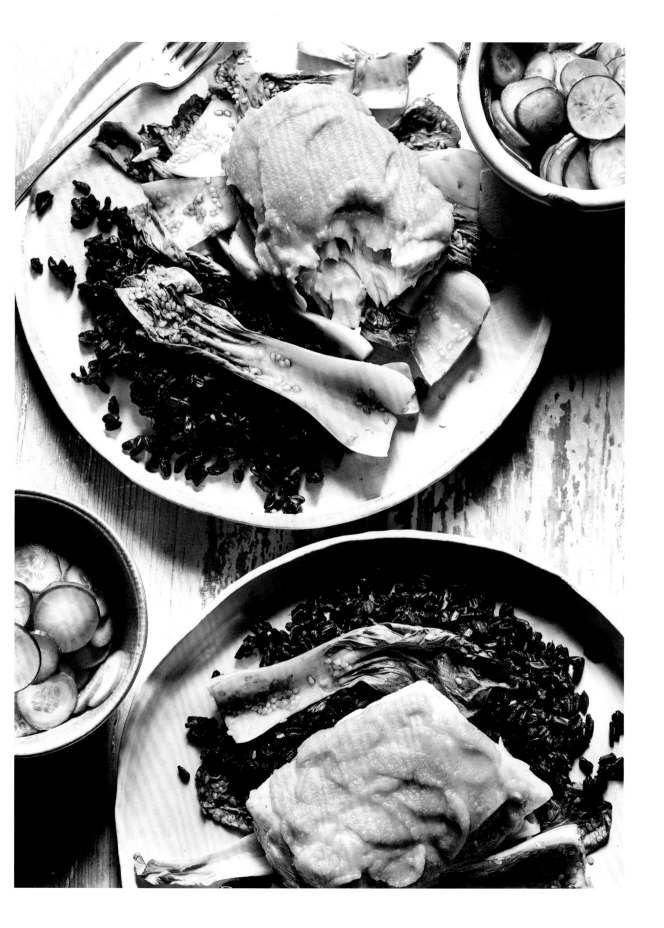

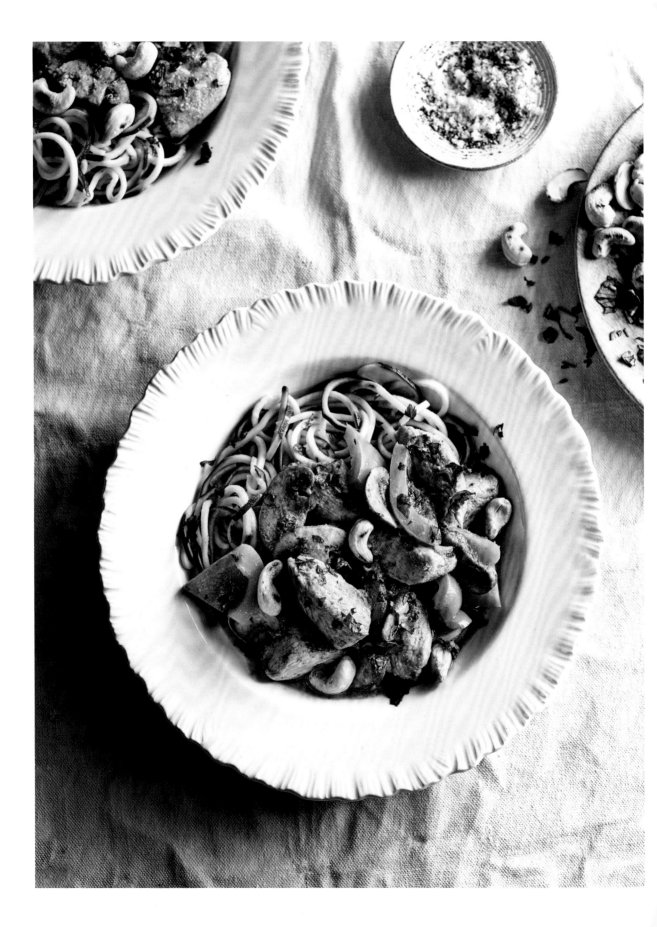

A dinner party favourite, this super-speedy red Thai chicken curry is so tasty that we know you'll make it again and again. Using the nutrient-packed courgetti instead of starchy white rice means you won't feel sluggish afterwards. For a heartier winter curry, we like to replace the orange pepper with oven-roasted butternut squash. To top this curry we've sprinkled over some cashew nuts, for added crunch and healthy fats.

RED THAI CHICKEN CURRY WITH COURGETTI & CASHEW NUTS

160g chestnut mushrooms
1 orange pepper
2 x 170g chicken breasts
handful of fresh coriander
coconut oil
1½ tbsp Thai red curry paste
200ml coconut milk
juice of 1 lime
300g courgettes
30g cashew nuts

1 Thinly slice the mushrooms and cut the orange pepper into bite-sized pieces. Slice the chicken breasts into bite-sized pieces. Roughly chop the coriander.

2 Heat ½ tablespoon of oil in a medium-sized pan on a medium heat. Add the red Thai curry paste and heat for 1 minute, then add the chicken, mix well to coat in the paste and cook for 5 minutes. Add the orange pepper and mushrooms and cook for 2 minutes.

3 Now add the coconut milk and simmer for 10 minutes, until the chicken is cooked through. Stir in half the coriander and half the lime juice.

4 While the curry is simmering, remove the ends of the courgettes, but leave the skin on. Peel the courgette into ribbons then slice the ribbons lengthways into long thin strips (or use a julienne peeler or spiraliser if you have one). Place in a bowl and mix in the rest of the lime juice.

5 Heat a dry frying pan and fry the cashew nuts for a few minutes, until lightly golden. Remove from the pan and set aside.

6 In the same frying pan, heat 1 teaspoon of oil and cook the courgetti for 2 minutes, stirring frequently.

7 Serve the curry in a bowl alongside a plate of courgetti noodles, or mix the two together. Garnish with the toasted cashew nuts and the remaining coriander.

We can't think of a better combination than creamy avocado and egg. In this recipe the egg is baked inside the avocado and is served alongside chicken sautéd in sun-dried tomato paste with a butternut squash mash. The sweetness of the squash is a perfect match for the richness of the dark leafy green cavolo nero. Cavolo nero (black kale), which originates from Tuscany, is a powerhouse of vitamins and minerals and like its popular cousin, curly kale, can help balance hormones.

SUN-DRIED TOMATO CHICKEN, SQUASH AND BAKED AVOCADO EGG

1 avocado
300g butternut squash
100g cavolo nero
2 sprigs of fresh basil
2 x 170g chicken breasts
2 eggs
olive oil
2 tbsp sun-dried tomato paste
sea salt and black pepper

1 Preheat the oven to 200°C/gas mark 6.

2 Cut the avocado in half and remove the stone. Peel the butternut squash and chop into 1cm cubes and thinly slice the cavolo nero. Finely chop the basil. Slice the chicken into thin strips.

3 Scoop out about 1 tablespoon from the centre of each avocado half to make space for an egg (snack on the middles as a cook's perk!). Crack one of the eggs into a bowl and slowly pour it into the centre of one of the avocado halves, then repeat with the other avocado half. Sprinkle with a pinch of sea salt, place on a baking tray and bake in the oven for 15 minutes, until the egg is cooked.

4 Meanwhile, place the squash in a saucepan with a pinch of sea salt and cover with boiling water. Boil for 7 minutes, then add the cavolo nero and boil for 3 minutes.

5 In a frying pan, heat ½ tablespoon of oil. Fry the chicken strips for 8–10 minutes, turning frequently, until cooked through, then season and stir in the sun-dried tomato paste, coating all the chicken.

6 Drain the squash and cavolo nero and mash gently together with a potato masher or the back of a fork. Mix in the chopped basil and season with sea salt and black pepper.

7 To serve, place the squash and cavolo nero mash on a plate, top with the sun-dried tomato chicken and place the avocado egg on the side.

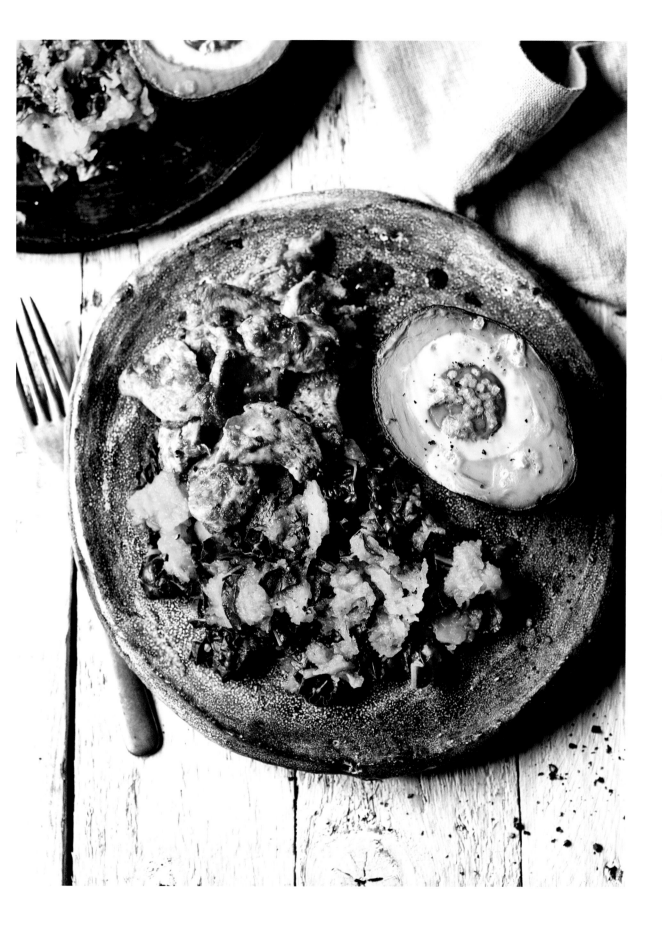

This healthy version of peanut satay sauce tastes amazing and is so simple to make. Peanuts are packed with good fats and are a great source of essential nutrients and vitamin E for heart health, while the fresh red chilli speeds up metabolism for a super-charged dish. We adore nutty black rice for its earthy flavour, satisfying texture and beneficial antioxidants – you can find it in health food stores or online, as well as some larger supermarkets.

PEANUT SATAY PORK WITH BLACK RICE, LEEK & RED PEPPER

80g black rice
400ml boiling water
2 tomatoes
1 leek
1 fresh red chilli
2 x 150g pork loin steaks
20g creamed coconut
2 tbsp peanut butter
2 tsp tamari
juice of ½ lime
coconut oil
80g spinach
sea salt

1 Rinse the black rice and put it into a pan with the boiling water and a pinch of sea salt. Simmer for 25–30 minutes, until the rice is cooked.

2 Meanwhile, cut each tomato into quarters. Slice the leek in half lengthways and chop into 2cm pieces, discarding the root. Finely chop the chilli. Slice the pork into thin strips.

3 To make the peanut satay sauce: in a bowl dissolve the creamed coconut with 2 tablespoons of boiling water, then stir in the peanut butter, tamari, red chilli and lime juice.

4 Heat ½ tablespoon of oil in a medium-sized pan on a medium-high heat and add the pork strips. Cook for 5 minutes, until browned, then add the leeks to the pan and cook for 3 minutes. Add the tomatoes and spinach and cook for a further 2 minutes.

5 Spoon the peanut satay sauce into the pan and cook for 2 minutes, until the pork is cooked through and the sauce has reduced slightly.

6 Drain the black rice.

7 To serve, place the black rice on a warm plate and spoon over the satay pork and vegetables.

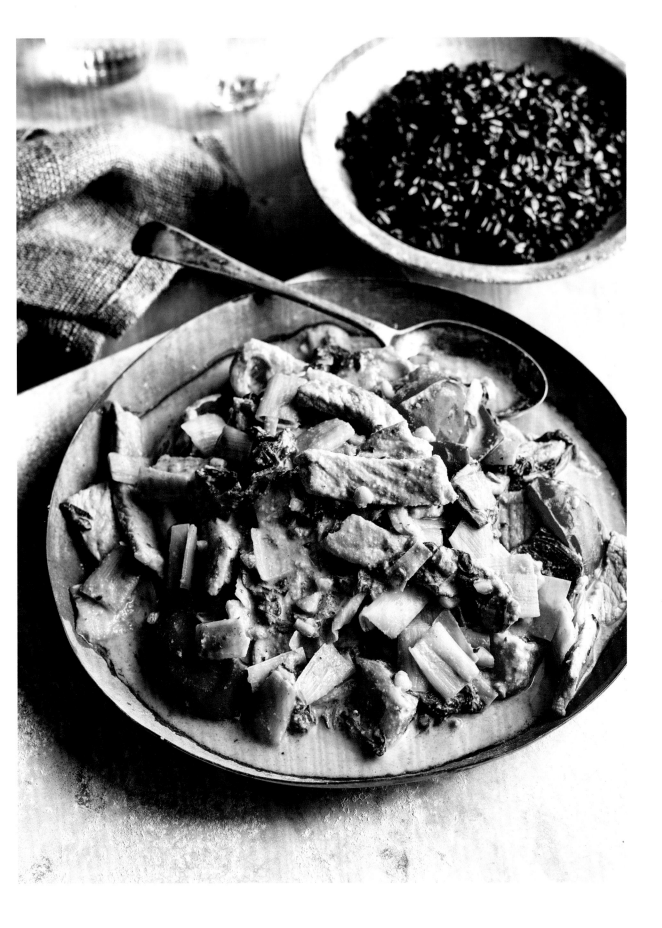

Lean pork loin is a delicious, healthy protein that contains minerals such as zinc and iron for energy release. The butter bean mash adds a creamy texture and soluble fibre for healthy digestion. Add more water or olive oil to the mash if it gets too dry, and season it well.

HONEY & MUSTARD PORK WITH BUTTER BEAN MASH & GREEN BEANS

120g green beans
handful of fresh flat-leaf parsley
1 tbsp wholegrain mustard
1½ tbsp honey
200g cherry tomatoes
olive oil
2 x 150g pork loin steaks
150g drained butter beans
100ml boiling water
sea salt and black pepper

1 Preheat the oven to 180°C/gas mark 4.

2 Trim the green beans and finely chop the parsley.

3 Mix the wholegrain mustard and honey in a small bowl.

4 Place the green beans and tomatoes on a baking tray. Drizzle over 1 teaspoon of oil and place in the oven for 10–15 minutes. When cooked, remove from the oven and keep warm.

5 Season both sides of the pork loin steaks with sea salt and black pepper. Heat ½ tablespoon of oil in a frying pan on a high heat, add the pork and fry for 5 minutes each side. Pour the honey and mustard sauce over the pork in the pan and cook for a further 3 minutes, until the meat is cooked through. Remove from the pan and leave to rest.

6 Meanwhile, put the drained butter beans into a saucepan with the boiling water and cook on a low heat for 5 minutes. Mash the beans with a potato masher or the back of a fork, then season and stir in the chopped parsley.

7 Thinly slice the pork. To serve, spoon the butter bean mash on to warm plates and place the pork slices on top. Serve with the roasted green beans and tomatoes.

The sweet and tangy balsamic vinegar glaze is a perfect match for a juicy steak. To accompany these rich flavours, we've made a butternut squash mash, lower in calories than mashed potato and a great source of beta-carotene, which keeps the heart healthy. We've upped the goodness in the mash with a hit of iron from the spinach to help transport oxygen around your body. This dish is sure to perk you up after a long day!

BALSAMIC & MUSTARD GLAZED BEEF WITH SQUASH & SPINACH MASH

140g cherry tomatoes
4 sprigs of fresh thyme
2 garlic cloves
100g chestnut mushrooms
400g butternut squash
olive oil
¼ beef stock cube
100ml boiling water
60g spinach
2 x 170g rump steaks
2 tbsp balsamic vinegar
1 tsp wholegrain mustard
sea salt and black pepper

1 Preheat the oven to 160°C/gas mark 3.

2 Halve the tomatoes and roughly chop the thyme leaves. Finely chop the garlic and finely slice the mushrooms. Peel the squash and cut it into 1cm pieces.

3 Place the tomatoes on a baking tray and drizzle over 1 teaspoon of oil. Cook in the oven for 15 minutes.

4 Dissolve the quarter stock cube in the boiling water.

5 Put the squash into a pan of boiling water and boil for 10 minutes, then add the spinach and simmer for a further 1 minute. Drain and mash with a potato masher (or the back of a fork).

6 Meanwhile, heat 2 teaspoons of oil in a frying pan. Season the steaks on both sides and place in the pan. Fry until golden brown: 2–3 minutes each side for medium rare or 4–5 minutes each side for well done. Remove the steaks from the pan and leave to rest.

7 Using the same frying pan on a medium heat, add 1 teaspoon of oil, the garlic and mushrooms and cook for 3 minutes, then add the balsamic vinegar, beef stock, mustard and thyme and cook for a further 3 minutes, until the sauce has reduced.

8 Cut the steaks into thin slices, arrange on plates, and spoon over the balsamic and mushroom sauce. Serve alongside the squash and spinach mash and the roasted tomatoes.

Fresh basil and garlic are a winning flavour combination, but they also have incredible health benefits. Basil aids digestion as well as containing a range of antioxidants, while garlic can help lower levels of insulin in the blood, reducing the risk of diabetes, and is even thought to aid weight loss. We've served these meatballs in a spicy tomato sauce, which has a deliciously smoky flavour from the chipotle paste.

BEEF MEATBALL & TOMATO BASIL RAGÙ WITH SQUASH NOODLES

2 garlic cloves
1 red onion
300g cherry tomatoes
a handful of fresh basil
300g butternut squash
olive oil
300g beef mince
80g spinach
2 tsp chipotle paste
sea salt and black pepper

1 Preheat the oven to 180°C/gas mark 4.

2 Finely chop or crush the garlic and finely slice the red onion. Cut the cherry tomatoes into quarters and finely slice the basil leaves.

3 Peel the butternut squash, then, using a peeler, slice the squash into long thin strips. Place the squash noodles on a baking tray, lightly toss in 1 tablespoon of oil, sprinkle with salt and place in the oven for 15 minutes.

4 Meanwhile, in a bowl, mix together the beef mince, garlic and half the basil leaves. Shape the mix into 8 balls.

5 Heat 1 teaspoon of oil in a frying pan on a medium-high heat and brown the meatballs on all sides for 10 minutes, until cooked through.

6 Meanwhile, heat 1 teaspoon of oil in another medium-sized pan. Fry the red onion for 5 minutes on a medium heat, then add the tomatoes, spinach and chipotle paste and cook for 5 minutes.

7 Remove the meatballs from the frying pan and add to the pan of tomatoes with the remaining basil. Place a lid on the pan and simmer for a further 5 minutes.

8 To serve, place the squash noodles on warm plates and spoon over the meatballs and tomato basil ragù.

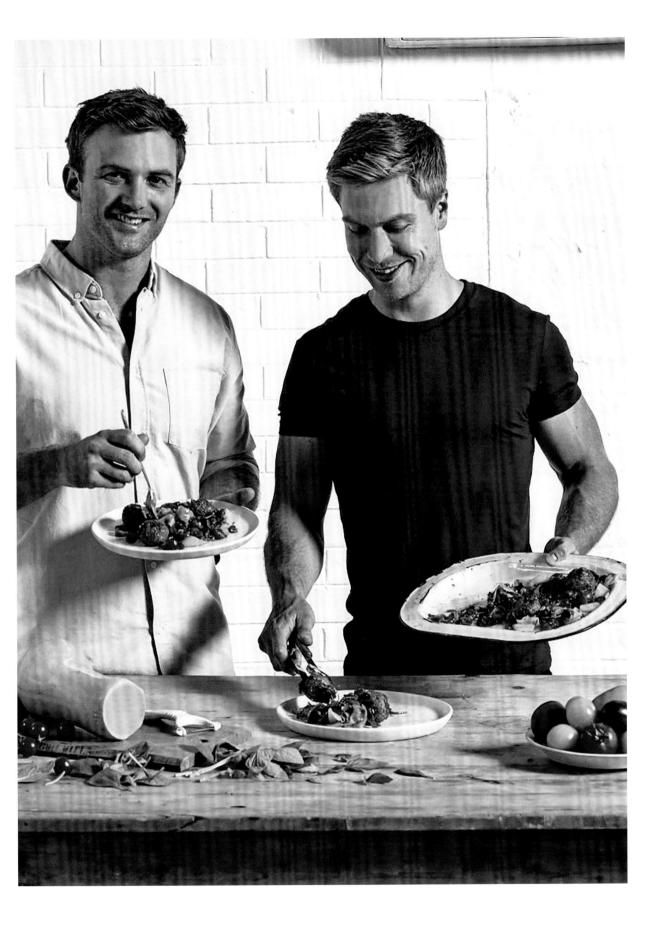

We've paired a succulent sirloin steak with a shaved asparagus and peppery rocket salad, drizzled with a balsamic glaze and an egg baked in a sweet potato. Sweet potatoes are slow-release carbohydrates that will leave you feeling not only fuller but also energised for longer. We boil the sweet potato first to speed up its cooking time.

SIRLOIN STEAK WITH SWEET POTATO BAKED EGG, BALSAMIC GLAZE & ASPARAGUS

1 sweet potato
100g asparagus
100g cherry tomatoes
40g rocket
olive oil
2 eggs
2 x 170g sirloin steaks
4 tbsp balsamic vinegar
15g pine nuts
sea salt and black pepper

1 Preheat the oven to 200°C/gas mark 6.

2 Cut the sweet potato in half lengthways, then place in a saucepan and cover with boiling water. Boil for 15 minutes, then drain and leave to cool for a few minutes.

3 Meanwhile, using a peeler, peel the asparagus into long thin ribbons. Cut the cherry tomatoes in half. Put the asparagus, tomatoes and rocket into a bowl with ½ tablespoon of olive oil and season.

4 Carefully remove a few tablespoons of sweet potato from the centre of each half. Crack an egg into each hole. Sprinkle with sea salt and place the sweet potatoes on a baking tray in the oven for 15 minutes, or until the egg white is set.

5 Heat ½ tablespoon of oil in a frying pan. Season the steaks on both sides and place in the pan. Cook until golden brown: 2–3 minutes each side for medium rare or 4–5 minutes each side for well done. Remove the steaks from the pan and leave to rest.

6 Heat a saucepan on a gentle heat. Pour in the balsamic vinegar and heat for 5 minutes, until the vinegar has reduced to a syrupy consistency.

7 Thinly slice the steaks and serve on warm plates, alongside the asparagus salad and sweet potato eggs. Drizzle the balsamic glaze over the salad and sprinkle over the pine nuts.

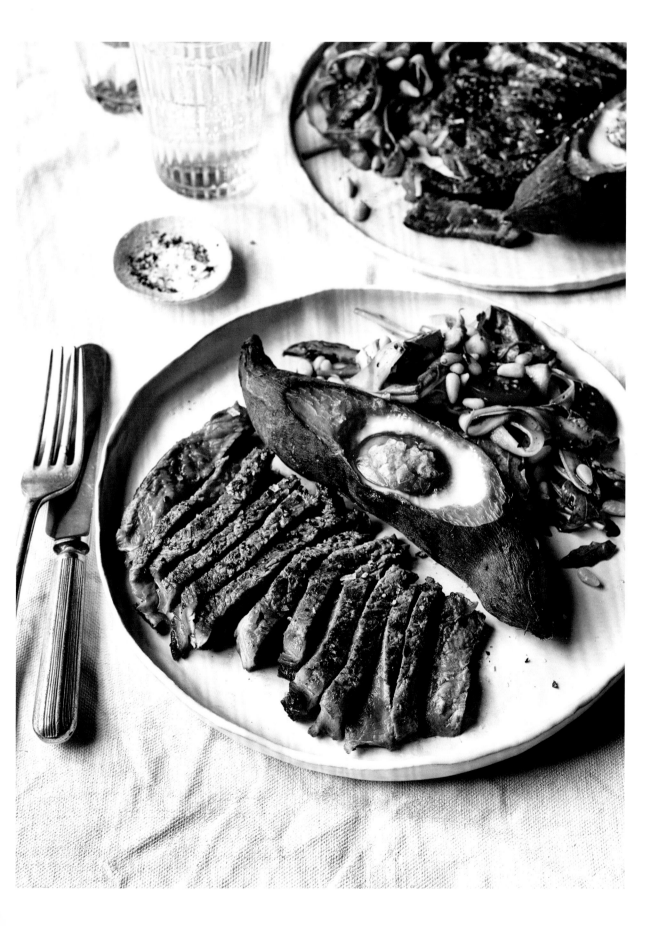

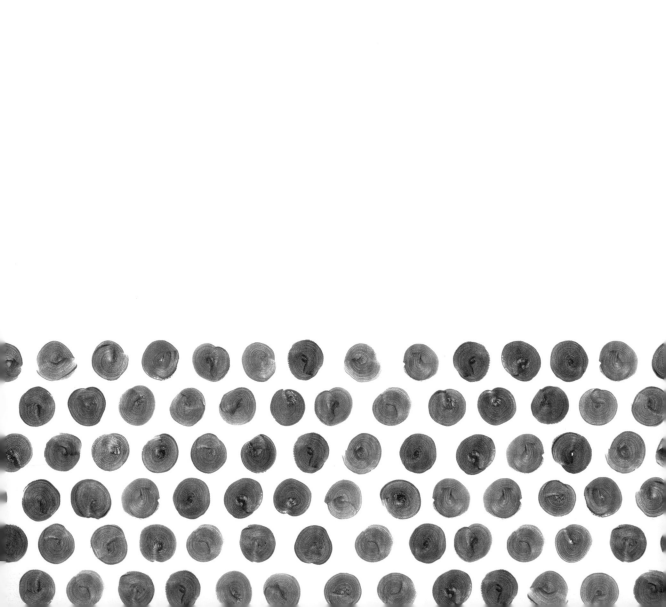

STRESS

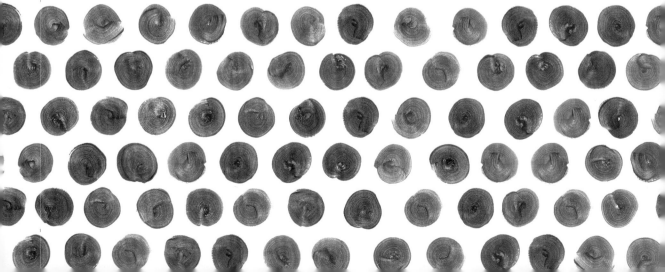

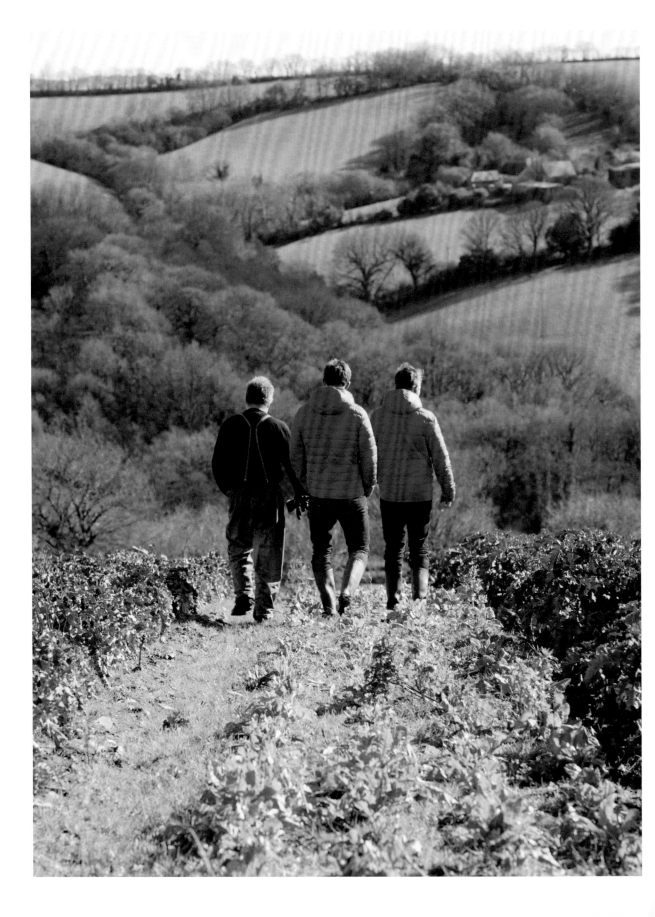

STRESS

The stress the modern person has to deal with is very different to that experienced by people millions of years ago. However, the way our bodies cope with stress has not changed. Our nervous system is the same and is hard-wired with two branches – the sympathetic nervous system and the parasympathetic nervous system. You may have heard of the sympathetic nervous system – it's often referred to as our fight or flight response. The parasympathetic nervous system is referred to as the rest and digest response. One activates a physiological response, while the other inhibits it. If you think back to our ancestors hunting and gathering the land, that fight or flight response would have been very appropriate, as they faced immediate dangers from animals or harsh environments. Today the threat of immediate danger for the average person is very rare, but our bodies are still hard-wired to react to stress in the same way.

And even though the problems we face are very different to those of our ancestors, we still have a lot to deal with on a daily basis. We stress over our jobs, our families, our financial stability – even commuting can be stressful.

There are two types of stress – good and bad. Good stress can come in various forms. An example of good stress is doing a bungee jump – even if this is something you've chosen to do and you enjoy it, it's still a stress on your body. Good stress is generally over quite quickly, but it can help keep us focused and energises us to tackle a problem head on. Many people are able to harness good stress and use it to their advantage. For example, someone in your office who is given a deadline may thrive on the time pressure, while another person in the same situation will hate it, worry about it and other areas of their work will suffer. This kind of 'bad stress' can be demotivating, negative and counterproductive.

In periods of stress the body is naturally wired to protect itself, so it triggers hormones to increase heart rate and blood pressure, to deliver oxygen and glucose to important muscles, and in turn it shuts down our non-critical functions. You may have heard of an ordinary person suddenly being able to lift a car up after a car accident, or performing other amazing feats of strength, and this is a direct response to the body shutting down non-urgent functions and prioritising physical functions so that it can either fight or escape (flight). In a life-threatening situation this is a great response and just what you need. However, in everyday life shutting down non-critical functions like our digestive system, liver metabolism and detoxification can be rather damaging. You can shut them down for intermittent periods but repeated shutdowns are not good for your body, as it creates imbalances. If you're constantly under stress, you're going to constantly stop these functions – they won't work optimally – which can lead to poor blood sugar management, depression, a reduced metabolism and muscle loss. If not managed properly, the result can be significant muscle loss, fat gain and hormonal imbalances.

Chronic stress also weakens the body by affecting the immune system. As you become more stressed, your immune system is put under attack, you become weaker and you can become ill as a result. It's one vicious cycle, and to fight it you need to ensure you are providing your body with the right type of nutrition to be able to act.

Regardless of your lifestyle, it is likely you are going to have to manage stress in some way and nutrition is one of the key ways to do this. There are certain foods you will want to avoid if you are overly stressed, as they will only serve to make you feel worse. Your basic ability to deal and manage the bad types of stress will also depend on a variety of factors, such as your personality type, your attitude and the people around you. There are many different ways to manage bad stress, and different means suit different people: meditation, yoga, sport, or simply planning how to deal with what's causing you stress are just a few examples, but by improving the types of food you are eating, and including foods that are full of the right vitamins and minerals, you can also help relieve some of the pressures faced by the body when it is stressed.

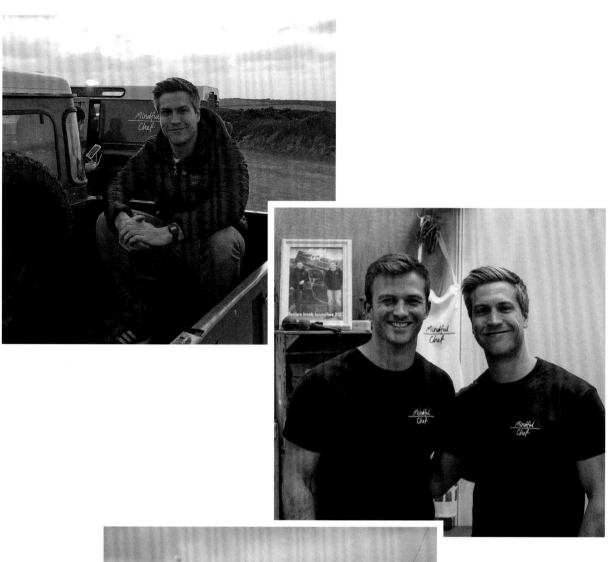

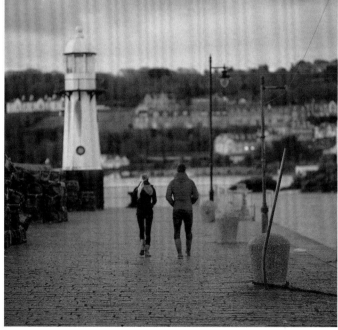

FOODS TO AVOID

- **SUGAR**
  Foods high in sugar can give an initial reprieve from stress as your energy is boosted. However, we know there is always an inevitable low following the high. We also know that when we are stressed we don't manage our blood sugar levels well. When we do crash we can become much more irritable and not nice to be around.

- **CAFFEINE**
  Caffeine actually reduces the body's ability to deal with stress. It acts as a stimulant and increases levels of cortisol, which is not good when you are stressed because your body has already increased cortisol as part of the fight or flight response.

- **PROCESSED FATS**
  Foods such as chocolate, chips, crisps, doughnuts should be avoided, as there is research to show that processed fat can increase levels of depression. This is obviously not good if you are also trying to deal with stress too.

- **ALCOHOL**
  Lots of people turn to alcohol as a coping mechanism. We've all reached for a beer or a glass of wine at the end of a long day. That's OK in moderation, but when it turns into several beers or a bottle of wine just as a means of escape, it becomes a problem. The side effects of alcohol are numerous, but addiction, sleep problems and nervousness are common.

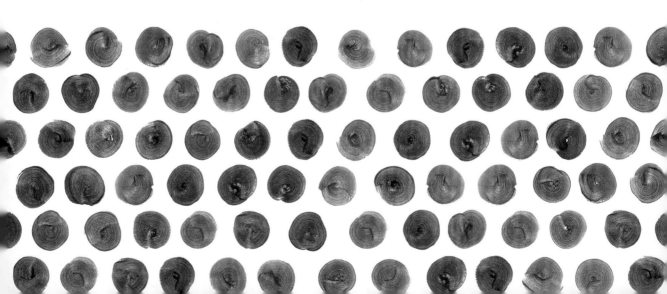

FOODS TO HELP MANAGE STRESS

- **ESSENTIAL FATTY ACIDS**
  Essential fatty acids, such as omega-3s can help moderate the effects of psychological and physical stress. You can find omega-3s in fish, pasture-raised animals, avocado, flax seeds and chia seeds.

- **B VITAMINS**
  Found in leafy greens, bananas, nuts and seeds, these vitamins help promote a working metabolism and keep blood cells healthy.

- **FRUIT AND VEGETABLES**
  These contain lots of nutrients and minerals that are crucial in helping the body when stressed.

- **VITAMIN C** The body's largest store of vitamin C is found in the adrenal glands. Adrenal fatigue, usually associated with high levels of stress, occurs when the body runs out of vitamin C and produces more cortisol (a steroid hormone that helps regulate energy in the body). More cortisol puts the body under more stress. If cortisol levels are high for a prolonged period it will affect your blood sugar levels and blood pressure management contribututing to the accumulation of belly fat. You may look and act fairly normal, but adrenal fatigue leads to general feelings of tiredness and low levels of energy. If you have to have a cup of coffee or energy drink in the morning in order to function, it's likely you may be suffering some form of adrenal fatigue. Keep your vitamin C stores full by eating lots of oranges, tomatoes, leafy greens and broccoli.

- **COMPLEX CARBOHYDRATES**
  These contain more nutrients than simple carbohydrates and are higher in fibre, meaning they will be digested more slowly. Think fruits, vegetables and wholegrain foods. Complex carbohydrates can help to enhance levels of serotonin – a mood-boosting hormone. You'll learn in chapter 5 how increased levels of sleep can help in the production of more serotonin, and eating the right types of food can help too: non-processed, wholegrain carbohydrates like the ones you will find in our recipes include brown rice and buckwheat.

- **GREEN TEA**
  Green tea contains L-theanine – a proven stress reducer. Green tea also helps by inhibiting cortisol, which the body releases in response to stress.

- **MAGNESIUM**
  This mineral helps the body relax and plays a vital role in hormone production, which is essential in keeping the body functioning while under stress. Foods containing magnesium include nuts, beans, lentils, whole grains and leafy greens.

TOP TIPS TO MANAGE YOUR STRESS LEVELS

1. **SPLIT TASKS DOWN INTO MANAGEABLE CHUNKS AND TACKLE THEM HEAD ON, ONE AT A TIME**
   You'll be far more productive and will get more done, rather than trying to do everything all at once and stressing yourself out.

2. **GET INTO A ROUTINE**
   Making yourself breakfast, lunch and dinner are all important times where you can completely zone out from what you are doing and have some you time. Plan when you are going to exercise and ensure that you are having enough sleep.

3. **PRACTISE MINDFUL TECHNIQUES SUCH AS PILATES, YOGA OR MEDITATION**
   It can even be as easy as just getting outside and enjoying nature.

4. **UNPLUG!**
   This is one of my biggest concerns for everyone. It is so hard for us to completely switch off and turn our backs on our phones, TV or the internet. But if you can plan to turn off your phone slightly earlier each evening, you will find there is time to concentrate on yourself more and on the things that really matter.

5. **NUTRITION IS KEY!**
   The type of food you are eating really can help reduce your stress levels. Not only do these foods help the body perform the vital functions it needs to while under stress, but they will also help you feel better in general. This could even stop the onset of stress, as you're able to manage it better.

For this chapter I have included some of my favourite recipes to help your body deal with stress. These meals include ingredients that are full of the vitamins and minerals listed on the previous page, all of which play a vital role in moderating the effects of physiological and psychological stress.

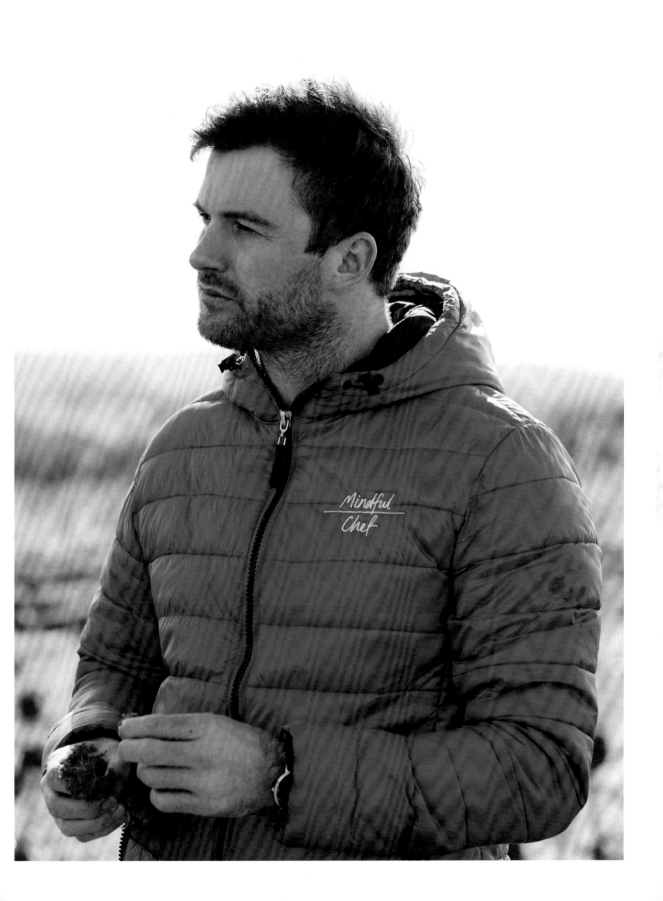

Lightly sautéd leek adds bite to these fritters, while chickpea flour binds the ingredients together. Tinned sweetcorn works well, but if you'd rather use a fresh ear of corn, try chargrilling it first, which will give the crispy fritters a satisfying smoky flavour.

SWEETCORN & LEEK FRITTERS WITH ROASTED TOMATOES & AVOCADO

2 garlic cloves

1 leek

coconut oil

140g asparagus

120g baby vine tomatoes

120g drained sweetcorn

6 tbsp chickpea flour

1 tsp smoked paprika

1 avocado

60g rocket

juice of 1 lime

sea salt and black pepper

1 Preheat the oven to 200°C/gas mark 6.

2 Finely chop or crush the garlic and finely slice the leek, discarding the root.

3 Heat ½ tablespoon of oil in a pan and fry the garlic and leeks for 5 minutes, until softened. Set aside.

4 Trim the asparagus. Place the cherry tomatoes and asparagus on a baking tray and drizzle with ½ tablespoon of oil and a pinch of sea salt. Bake in the oven for 10 minutes.

5 Meanwhile, drain the sweetcorn. In a bowl, mix the sweetcorn, chickpea flour and smoked paprika with the softened leeks and garlic. Add 2–3 tablespoons of cold water and season with sea salt and black pepper. Form the mixture into 6 fritters, each about 1cm thick.

6 Heat 1 tablespoon of oil in a large frying pan on a medium–high heat and fry the fritters for 3–4 minutes on each side, until golden brown.

7 Meanwhile, peel and de-stone the avocado and cut into thick slices.

8 To serve, place the rocket on plates, arrange the sweetcorn and leek fritters on top, and serve alongside the sliced avocado, roasted asparagus and tomatoes. Drizzle over the juice from the lime.

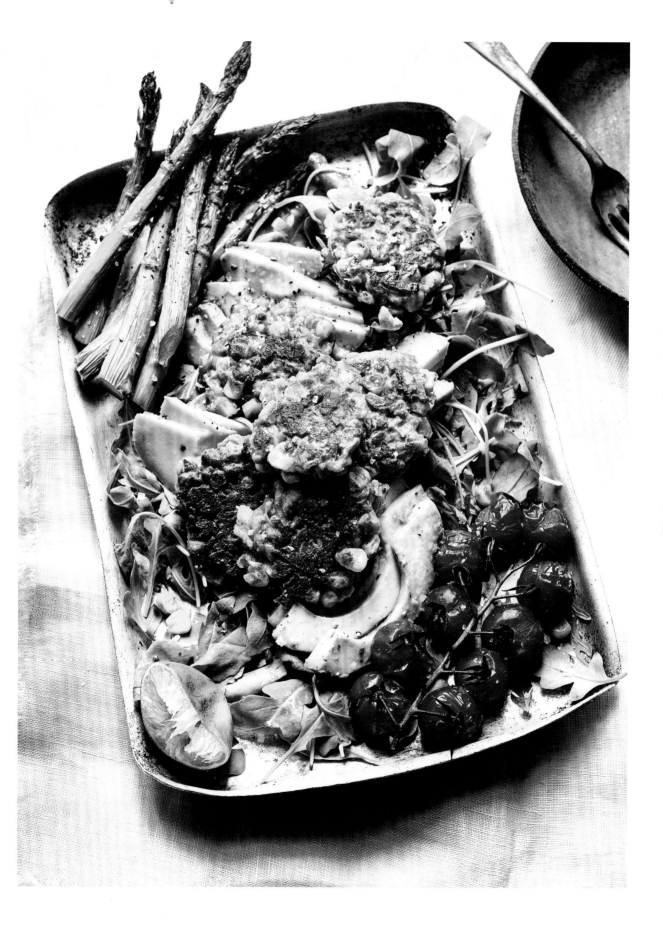

We've created a superfood pizza, made with buckwheat flour and omega-3 loaded chia seeds. As well as being packed with nutritional benefits, when soaked in water chia seeds act like an egg, binding dry ingredients together. We've topped this protein-packed pizza base with chunky basil-infused hummus, griddled courgette slices, creamy avocado and tangy balsamic onions.

BUCKWHEAT CHIA PIZZA WITH HUMMUS & CHARGRILLED COURGETTE

2 tbsp chia seeds
1 garlic clove
1 red onion
150g courgettes
1 avocado
150g buckwheat flour
120g drained chickpeas
olive oil
handful of fresh basil
2 tbsp balsamic vinegar
60g rocket
sea salt and black pepper

1 Preheat the oven to 180°C/gas mark 4.

2 In a bowl, mix the chia seeds with 6 tablespoons of cold water and leave for 5 minutes.

3 Finely chop the garlic. Thinly slice the red onion and cut the courgettes into long thin strips. Peel and de-stone the avocado and thinly slice.

4 Mix the buckwheat flour with the chia seeds, a pinch of sea salt and 8 tablespoons of cold water to form a dough. Halve the dough and spread out on a sheet of baking paper into a pizza shape 15cm in diameter. Repeat with the remaining dough. Bake the two pizzas in the oven for 15 minutes.

5 Meanwhile, drain the chickpeas and put them into a bowl with the garlic, 2 teaspoons of oil and 2 tablespoons of cold water. Season with salt and pepper, then mash the chickpeas with a potato masher until they are all crushed. Finely slice the basil and stir into the hummus.

6 Heat 1 teaspoon of oil in a frying pan on a medium heat and fry the red onion for 5 minutes. Add half the balsamic vinegar and cook for a further 3 minutes, then turn off the heat.

7 Drizzle the courgette strips with 1 teaspoon of oil. Heat a griddle pan on a medium heat and cook the courgette strips for 2–3 minutes each side. Spread the basil hummus over the pizza, and top with the courgette, balsamic onions and avocado. Drizzle over the remaining balsamic vinegar and serve with the rocket alongside.

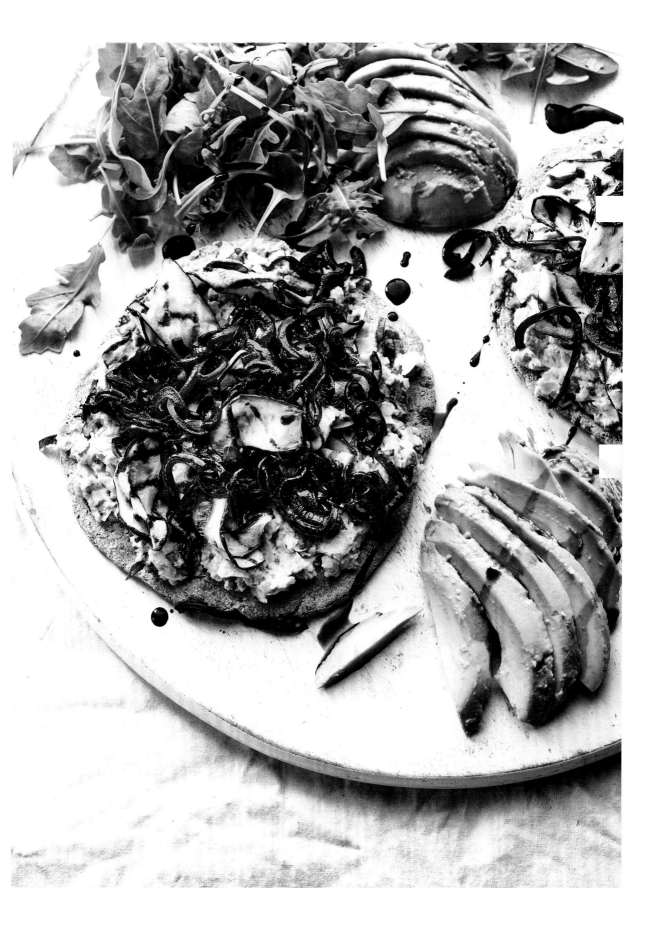

This creamy and fragrant beef curry is a quick and easy version of the Indonesian classic. Cinnamon is one of the oldest known spices, and contains a wealth of health-giving properties from soothing muscles to stimulating circulation. Fresh lemongrass brings a light citrus flavour and has long been regarded for its medicinal properties, including its anti-inflammatory benefits. The oil from lemongrass can even be used topically and in aromatherapy to help treat aches and pains.

BEEF RENDANG WITH LEMONGRASS, MANGETOUT & BROWN RICE

80g brown rice
400ml boiling water
2 garlic cloves
4cm fresh ginger
1 fresh lemongrass stalk
1 fresh red chilli
80g baby sweetcorn
80g mangetout
handful of fresh coriander
2 x 170g centre cut beef steaks
coconut oil
200ml coconut milk
½ tsp ground cinnamon
sea salt

1 Rinse the brown rice, then put it into a saucepan with the boiling water and a pinch of sea salt and simmer for 20–25 minutes, until cooked.

2 Peel and finely chop the garlic and ginger. Trim the ends of the lemongrass, remove the outer layer and finely chop. Thinly slice the red chilli.

3 Trim the baby sweetcorn and mangetout. Roughly chop the coriander. Cut the beef into bite-sized chunks.

4 Heat 1 tablespoon of oil in a medium-sized pan on a medium heat and fry the garlic, ginger, chilli and lemongrass for 2 minutes. Then add the beef and cook for 7 minutes, until browned.

5 Add the baby sweetcorn, coconut milk and cinnamon and simmer for 5 minutes, then add the mangetout and cook for a further 5 minutes, until the sauce has reduced. Season with a pinch of sea salt.

6 Drain the brown rice and stir in the coriander.

7 Serve the rice on a warm plate, make a well in the centre and spoon over the beef rendang.

Many meat-eaters avoid tofu, thinking it's a bland and boring alternative to meat, but we're here to assure you tofu can be fantastically tasty. It absorbs flavours like a sponge so you can pack it with as much punch and taste as you like. Here we've partnered it with a moreish peanut sauce, pepped up with fresh lime and red chilli.

TOFU PAD THAI WITH CRUNCHY PEANUTS & COURGETTE NOODLES

1 fresh red chilli
4 spring onions
200g carrots
1 yellow pepper
handful of fresh coriander
300g courgettes
300g firm tofu
coconut oil
2 tbsp tamari
2 tbsp peanut butter
2 tsp maple syrup
juice of 2 limes

1 Finely chop the chilli and finely slice the spring onions, removing the root at the end. Slice the carrots into matchsticks, and thinly slice the yellow pepper. Roughly chop the coriander leaves.

2 Remove the ends of the courgettes, but leave the skin on. Prepare the courgetti noodles by peeling them into ribbons, then slicing these lengthways into thin strips (or use a julienne peeler or spiraliser if you have one).

3 Drain the tofu, then rinse and chop into 2cm cubes. Pat dry with kitchen paper.

4 Heat 1 tablespoon of oil in a pan and fry the tofu for 5 minutes, then add half the tamari and fry for another 5 minutess until golden brown, turning occasionally.

5 Meanwhile, to make the sauce, mix the peanut butter with the remaining tamari, the maple syrup, half the lime juice and the chilli.

6 Heat 1 tablespoon of oil in another pan and fry the carrot, spring onion and yellow pepper for 2 minutes. Then add the courgette noodles, half the coriander and the sauce and cook for 3 minutes.

7 Serve the pad Thai in warm bowls, top with the tofu and sprinkle over the remaining coriander leaves and lime juice.

This is our favourite fish pie – so creamy yet without any dairy. You'll notice that throughout the book we often use coconut milk as a replacement for milk or cream – it has a similar texture and is full of beneficial fats. The hot-smoked salmon is not only incredibly tasty, it's a such a useful ingredient for the time-poor: it's ready to eat so it can be added towards the end of cooking, just to heat through. Carrots make a lighter, vibrant version of the traditional potato topping.

HOT SMOKED SALMON & COCONUT FISH PIE WITH CARROT MASH

400g carrots
120g green beans
1 leek
handful of fresh flat-leaf parsley
olive oil
200ml coconut milk
2 tsp cornflour
1 tsp wholegrain mustard
300g hot-smoked salmon
80g spinach
sea salt and black pepper

1 Peel the carrots and chop them into 1cm rounds. Trim the green beans and thinly slice the leek, removing the root end. Roughly chop the parsley.

2 Place the carrots in a saucepan of boiling water and simmer with a pinch of sea salt for 20 minutes, until soft. In the last 5 minutes, add the green beans. Drain the vegetables, remove the green beans and keep warm, then mash the carrot with a potato masher (or with a fork).

3 Meanwhile, heat 1 teaspoon of oil in a medium-sized pan and fry the leek for 5 minutes.

4 Pour 2 tablespoons of the coconut milk into a bowl and mix in the cornflour to form a smooth paste. Add the remaining coconut milk to the leek pan with the cornflour mix and the mustard and simmer gently for 10 minutes, until the sauce thickens.

5 Preheat the grill to high. Break the salmon into pieces, stir it into the coconut sauce with the spinach and half the parsley and cook for 2 minutes. Season with sea salt and black pepper.

6 Place the fish pie mix in an ovenproof dish and spoon over the carrot mash. Place under the grill for 5 minutes.

7 Scatter over the remaining parsley and serve the pie with the green beans alongside.

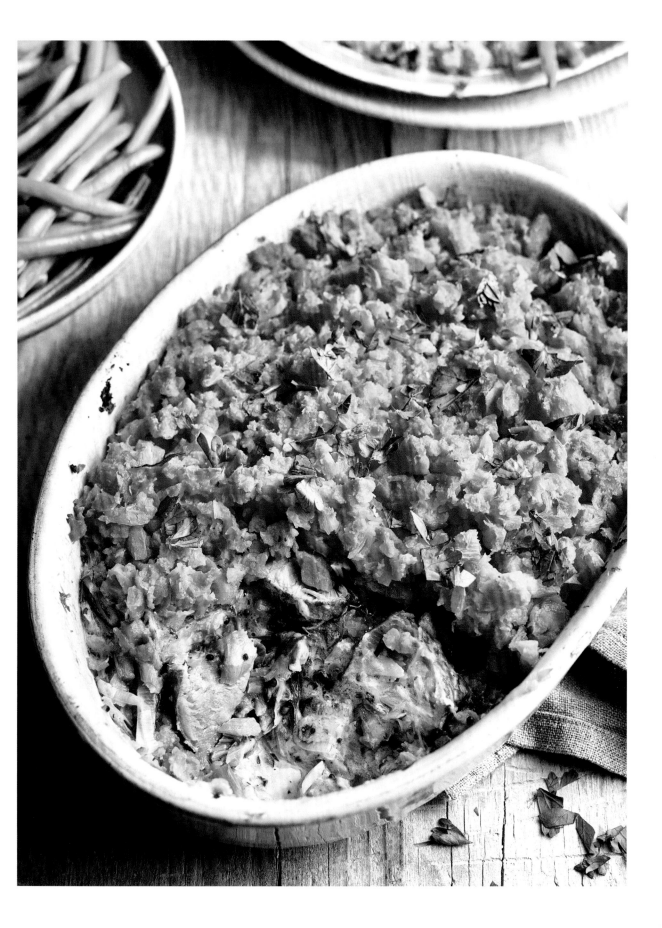

Fajitas don't have to be made with wheat flour – you can make protein-packed buckwheat wraps quickly and easily at home in less time than it would take to pop out to your local shop. They need a good seasoning of salt and pepper, and you could always add a bit of smoked paprika too.

PAPRIKA HADDOCK BUCKWHEAT FAJITAS WITH COCONUT DRIZZLE

2 tomatoes
4 spring onions
1 gem lettuce
100g carrots
80g buckwheat flour
coconut oil
240g drained black beans
½ tsp chilli flakes
2 tsp smoked paprika
300g haddock fillets
20g creamed coconut
20ml boiling water
juice of 1 lime
sea salt and black pepper

1 Dice the tomatoes and finely slice the spring onions. Roughly slice the gem lettuce, removing the root end. Grate the carrot.

2 To make two fajitas: in a bowl, mix the buckwheat flour with 150ml of cold water, ½ tablespoon of oil and a pinch of sea salt, until a smooth batter is formed.

3 In a large frying pan, heat 1 teaspoon of oil on a medium heat. Pour in half the buckwheat mix to form a large thin pancake and cook for 3 minutes each side, until turning golden, then remove from the pan and keep warm. Repeat with the remaining batter.

4 Heat 1 teaspoon of oil in a medium-sized frying pan on a medium heat and cook the spring onions for 2 minutes. Add the drained beans, tomatoes, chilli flakes and half the paprika, then season with salt and pepper and cook for 7 minutes.

5 Meanwhile, slice the haddock into small pieces. Place in a bowl with the rest of the paprika, a pinch of sea salt and ½ tablespoon of oil, and mix well. In a frying pan, fry the fish for 6–8 minutes on a medium heat, until cooked through.

6 In a bowl, dissolve the creamed coconut in the boiling water.

7 Place the fajitas on plates and top with the lettuce, carrot and beans, followed by the haddock. Drizzle with the coconut and squeeze over the lime juice.

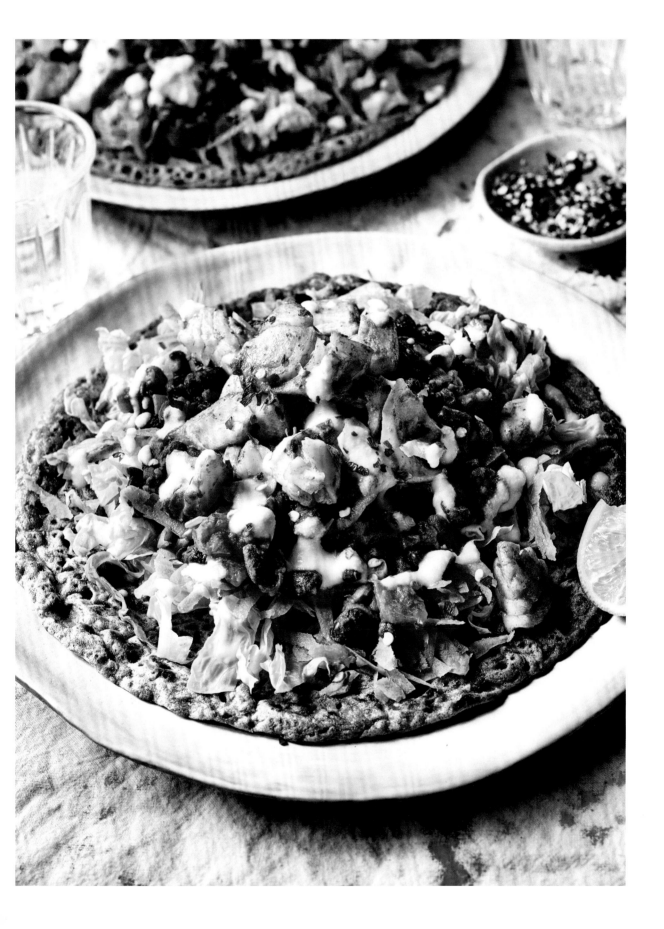

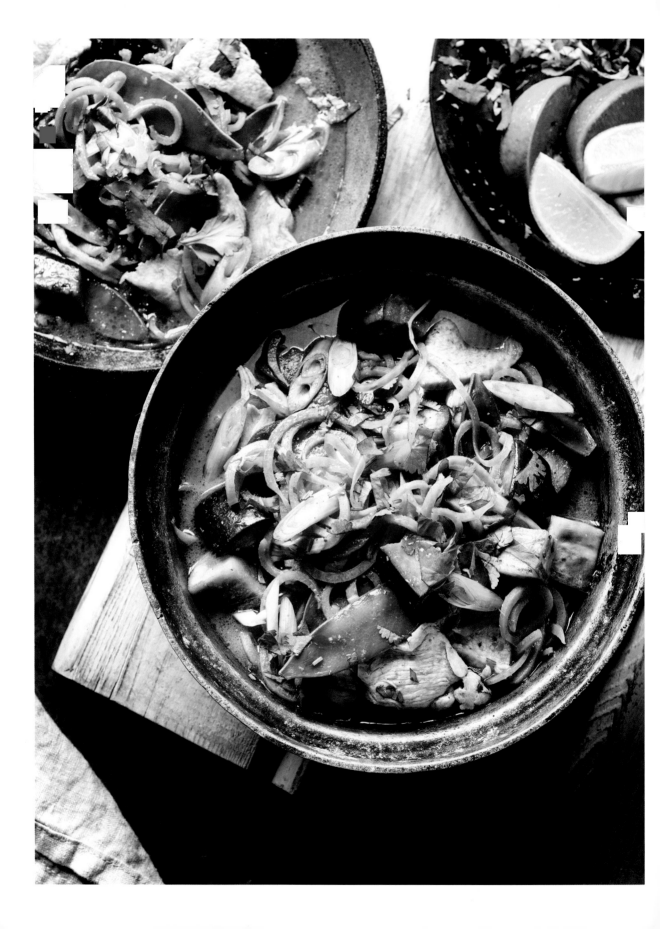

Tom yum soup is a hot spicy broth from Thailand, but in this version we add coconut milk to temper the heat from the chilli. The spice paste includes lemongrass, galangal (a root from the ginger family), garlic and chilli, and we've paired its fragrant flavour with aubergine, mangetout and carrot noodles. Carrots contain beta-carotene, which the body transforms into a usuable source of vitamin A, associated with protection against cardiovascular disease.

SPICY TOM YUM CHICKEN & COCONUT SOUP WITH CARROT NOODLES

4 spring onions
1 aubergine
handful of fresh coriander
300g chicken breasts
280g carrots
coconut oil
80g mangetout
1 vegetable stock cube
300ml boiling water
200ml coconut milk
2 tsp tom yum paste
juice of 1 lime

1 Finely slice the spring onions and cut the aubergine into 2cm cubes. Roughly chop the coriander. Thinly slice the chicken breasts.

2 Peel the carrots. Slice the carrot into long thin strips using a peeler, julienne peeler or spiraliser if you have one.

3 In a frying pan, heat ½ tablespoon of oil on a medium heat and fry the aubergine for 5 minutes, until softened. Remove from the pan and set aside.

4 In the same pan, heat another ½ tablespoon of oil on a medium heat. Add the chicken and cook for 8 minutes, until golden brown. Add the spring onions and mangetout and fry for 2 minutes, until the chicken is cooked through.

5 Meanwhile, put the stock cube into a separate pan with the boiling water and stir until dissolved. Add the coconut milk and stir in the tom yum paste. Bring to the boil, then stir in the cooked chicken, mangetout, spring onions, aubergine, carrot noodles and the juice of the lime. Simmer for 3 minutes.

6 Serve the soup in warm bowls and sprinkle over the coriander.

Buckwheat, despite its misleading name, does not actually contain wheat and is naturally gluten free. It has a lovely nutty texture and contains all eight essential amino acids, plus it is rich in magnesium, which helps regulate blood sugar levels. In this recipe we've mixed buckwheat with ripe tomatoes, red pepper and sweetcorn for a refreshing side to the spicy jerk chicken. We've butterflied the chicken breasts so they cook in half the time.

BUTTERFLIED CHARGRILLED JERK CHICKEN WITH SWEETCORN & BUCKWHEAT

80g buckwheat
400ml boiling water
2 x 180g chicken breasts
coconut oil
1 tbsp jerk seasoning
½ red onion
2 tomatoes
1 fresh green chilli
juice of 1 lime
1 red pepper
handful of fresh coriander
100g drained sweetcorn
sea salt and black pepper

1 Rinse the buckwheat and place it in a saucepan with the boiling water, then simmer for 15 minutes.

2 To butterfly the chicken, carefully slice through one side of each breast from the thickest part to the thinnest, being careful not to cut right through to the end. Open out each chicken breast to resemble a butterfly. Place in a bowl with 1 tablespoon of oil, the jerk seasoning and a pinch of sea salt.

3 Heat a griddle pan (or barbecue) to a medium–high heat. Add the butterflied chicken breasts and cook for 5–10 minutes each side, or until the chicken is cooked through.

4 While the chicken is cooking, make the chilli tomato salsa: finely dice the red onion and tomatoes and finely chop the chilli. Mix together in a bowl with half the lime juice.

5 Dice the red pepper, roughly chop the coriander and drain the sweetcorn. Drain the cooked buckwheat and stir in the red pepper, sweetcorn and half the coriander. Season with sea salt and black pepper.

6 Spoon the buckwheat on to plates, top with the chicken, and serve the salsa alongside. Sprinkle the chicken with the remaining coriander leaves and drizzle over the rest of the lime juice.

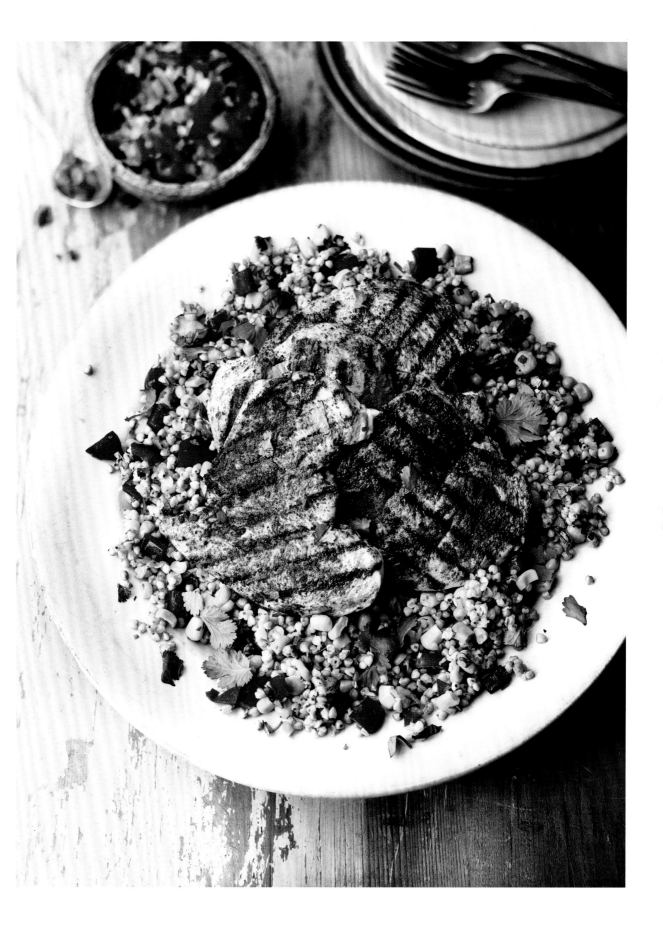

This summery Spanish-style roasted chicken thigh paella is made with the ancient grain quinoa, instead of with starchy rice. Originally from the Andes mountains in South America, quinoa is a nutritious alternative to refined carbohydrates, as it contains all eight essential amino acids, as well as being loaded with vitamins.

CHICKEN & QUINOA PAELLA WITH ARTICHOKES, OLIVES & LEMON

½ a chicken stock cube
300ml boiling water
2 garlic cloves
1 orange pepper
100g cherry tomatoes
handful of fresh flat-leaf parsley
1 lemon
4 chicken thighs, skinless
    and boneless
2 tsp smoked paprika
olive oil
80g quinoa
60g pitted black olives
80g drained artichoke hearts in
    brine
sea salt and black pepper

1 Preheat the oven to 200°C/gas mark 6.

2 Dissolve the stock cube in the boiling water.

3 Finely chop the garlic and thinly slice the orange pepper. Halve the cherry tomatoes and roughly chop the parsley leaves. Cut the lemon in half, keep half for the juice and chop the remaining half into 4 wedges.

4 Place the chicken thighs on a baking tray or in an ovenproof dish. Season them with sea salt and black pepper, a quarter of the smoked paprika and drizzle with ½ tablespoon of oil. Place in the oven for 20 minutes, or until the chicken is cooked through.

5 Meanwhile, heat ½ tablespoon of oil in a medium-sized pan on a medium heat. Add the garlic and cook for 2 minutes. Rinse the quinoa and add to the pan with the chicken stock, remaining paprika and the orange pepper, then simmer for 10 minutes with the lid on.

6 Remove the lid, stir in the tomatoes, olives, artichokes and reserved lemon juice and simmer for a further 5 minutes, until all the liquid has been absorbed. Add more boiling water if needed. Stir in half the parsley and season with black pepper.

7 To serve, spoon the paella into warm bowls, top with the chicken and scatter over the remaining parsley. Serve with the lemon wedges.

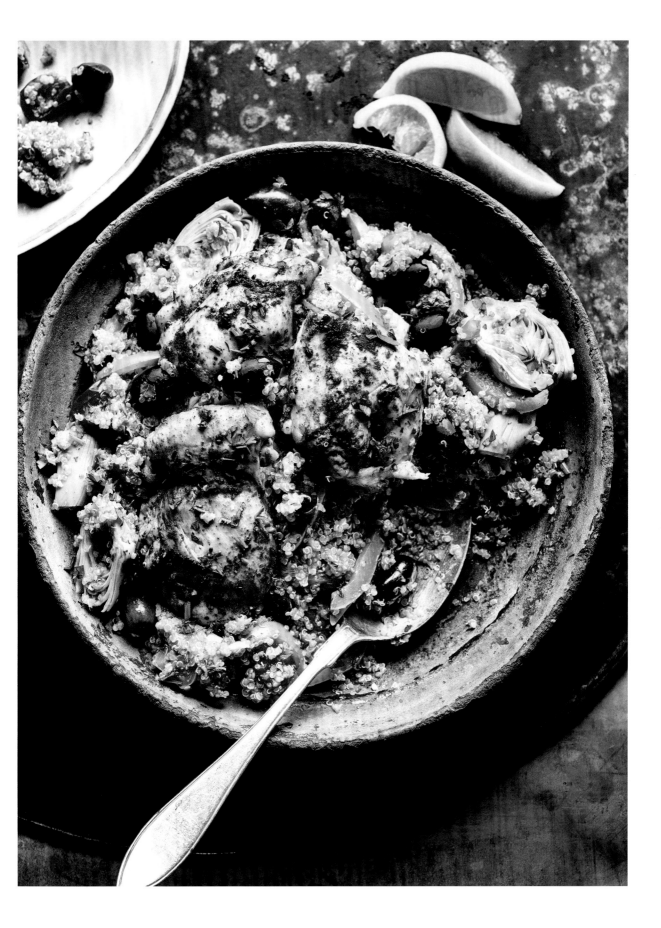

We've used pork instead of the more traditional beef in this chilli recipe, for its rich flavour and to complement the smokiness of the paprika wedges. Smooth, buttery avocado and lime juice add a cooling zingy textural contrast. We include lots of avocado in our diet for its creamy flavour and its omega-3 fatty acids, which enhance brain function. If you can get your hands on avocado oil too, this makes a really tasty dressing for salads and can help fight free radicals.

PORK CHILLI WITH PAPRIKA SWEET POTATO WEDGES & AVOCADO

2 garlic cloves
1 red onion
olive oil
300g sweet potatoes
2 tsp smoked paprika
300g pork mince
1 tsp chilli flakes
200g passata
1 avocado
handful of fresh coriander
juice of 1 lime
sea salt and black pepper

1 Preheat the oven to 200°C/gas mark 6.

2 Finely chop or crush the garlic. Finely slice the red onion.

3 Heat 1 teaspoon of oil in a medium-sized pan on a medium heat and fry the garlic and red onion for 5 minutes, until softened.

4 Meanwhile, slice the sweet potato into small wedges. Toss the wedges with ½ tablespoon of oil, half the paprika and a pinch of salt. Spread out on a baking tray and bake in the oven for 20 minutes, turning halfway through the cooking time.

5 Add the pork mince to the pan of red onion and cook for 10 minutes, until golden, breaking the mince up in the pan. Add the chilli flakes, the remaining paprika and the passata and cook for a further 10 minutes, until the sauce has thickened. Season with salt and pepper.

6 Peel and de-stone the avocado, then thinly slice. Roughly chop the coriander.

7 Spoon the pork chilli on to warm plates, sprinkle over the coriander and serve alongside the sweet potato wedges and avocado alongside. Drizzle over the lime juice.

Don't be put off by celeriac's strange bulbous look – it's such a versatile vegetable and is loaded with B vitamins. Peeled and grated, it has a delicate celery flavour which is delicious in this raw slaw with Dijon mustard, fresh thyme, olive oil and lemon juice. The crispy sage adds a satisfying crunch alongside the soft roasted pears and tender pork. We recommend using English Conference pears – if you aren't able to find ripe pears, increase the cooking time slightly.

ROAST PORK & PEAR WITH CRISPY SAGE, TENDERSTEM & CELERIAC SLAW

1 pear
200g tenderstem broccoli
2–3 sprigs of fresh thyme
2–3 sprigs of fresh sage
2 x 150g pork loin steaks
olive oil
juice of ½ lemon
1 tsp Dijon mustard
200g celeriac
sea salt and black pepper

1 Preheat the oven to 200°C/gas mark 6.

2 Cut the pear in half, remove the core, then slice each half into 6 thin wedges. Trim the tenderstem. Remove the thyme and sage leaves from their stalks.

3 Season the pork with salt and pepper. Heat ½ tablespoon of oil in a frying pan on a medium heat and fry the pork for 2–3 minutes each side, until golden brown.

4 Put the pork on a baking tray and place the tenderstem and pear slices alongside. Drizzle with ½ tablespoon of oil and scatter over half the thyme leaves. Place in the oven and cook for 10 minutes, or until the meat is cooked through.

5 In a bowl, mix the lemon juice, mustard, ½ tablespoon of olive oil and the remaining thyme leaves, then season with sea salt and black pepper. Peel and grate the celeriac and add to the bowl, stirring to coat in the dressing.

6 In the same frying pan as before, heat 1 teaspoon of oil on a medium heat and fry the sage leaves for 3 minutes, until turning crispy.

7 Place the pork on warm plates and top with the sliced pear and crispy sage. Serve the tenderstem and celeriac slaw alongside.

Inspired by the traditional souvlaki of Greece, our tender lamb skewers are marinated in a mix of fresh garlic, ground cumin and dried oregano and can be chargrilled in a griddle pan or on a barbecue. We serve our skewers with roasted sweet potatoes and a refreshing Greek-style salad packed with black olives. Olives and olive oil have many nutritional benefits, including oleic acid, an omega-9 fatty acid, great for soothing the skin, and high levels of good cholesterol for lowering the risk of heart disease.

LAMB SOUVLAKI WITH GREEK-STYLE SALAD & ROASTED SWEET POTATOES

2 garlic cloves
1 tsp ground cumin
2 tsp dried oregano
olive oil
300g diced lamb shoulder
300g sweet potato
1 baby cucumber
2 tomatoes
40g black pitted olives
a few sprigs of fresh mint
1 tbsp white wine vinegar
sea salt and black pepper

1 Preheat the oven to 200°C/gas mark 6.

2 Finely chop or crush the garlic. To make the marinade, mix the cumin, half the oregano, the garlic and 1 tablespoon of olive oil in a bowl and season with sea salt and black pepper.

3 Place the diced lamb in the bowl, coat with the marinade and leave for 10 minutes.

4 Meanwhile, peel the sweet potato and dice into 1cm cubes. Toss with 1 teaspoon of oil and the remaining oregano, then place on a baking tray and roast for 15–20 minutes, turning halfway through.

5 Thread the lamb on to four skewers.

6 Preheat a griddle pan (or barbecue) on a medium-high heat. Add the skewers and cook for 10–15 minutes, turning every 2–3 minutes, until all sides are golden brown and the lamb is cooked through.

7 To make the Greek-style salad: dice the cucumber and tomatoes, halve the black olives, and finely slice the mint. Place in a bowl with 2 teaspoons of olive oil and the white wine vinegar and season with salt and pepper.

8 Divide the salad between serving plates, alongside the roasted sweet potatoes, and top each one with 2 skewers.

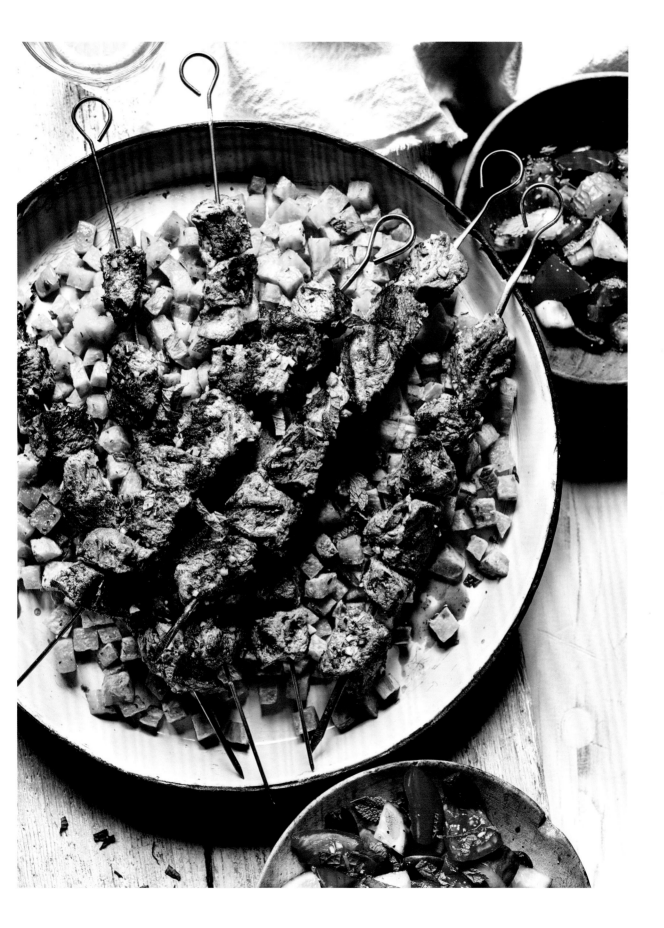

This dish is inspired by the vibrant flavours of Persian cuisine. The lamb is marinated in sticky, sweet pomegranate molasses and spiced with ground cumin, while the quinoa is studded with fresh pomegranate seeds, which are packed with powerful antioxidants and loaded with vitamin C. We've drizzled over tahini, which is simply ground toasted sesame seeds, rich in minerals such as magnesium and potassium. It is also an excellent source of calcium, so it's particularly good if you are avoiding dairy.

PERSIAN LAMB WITH AUBERGINE, POMEGRANATE & MINT QUINOA

80g quinoa
300ml boiling water
½ pomegranate
1 baby cucumber
handful of fresh mint
1 aubergine
2 tbsp pomegranate molasses
juice of 1 lemon
1 tsp ground cumin
olive oil
2 x 150g lamb leg steaks
2 tsp tahini
sea salt

1 Rinse the quinoa and place it in a pan with the boiling water and a pinch of sea salt. Simmer for 15–20 minutes, until the quinoa is cooked.

2 Meanwhile, remove the seeds from the pomegranate half. Slice the cucumber into thin half-moons and roughly chop the mint leaves. Slice the aubergine into thin rounds.

3 In a bowl, mix half the pomegranate molasses with half the lemon juice, the cumin, a pinch of sea salt and 1 teaspoon of oil. Rub this mixture over both sides of the lamb steaks. Heat 1 teaspoon of oil in a frying pan on a medium heat and fry the lamb steaks for 4–5 minutes on each side, until cooked. Remove from the pan and leave to rest for 5 minutes.

4 Heat 1 teaspoon of oil in the same pan and cook the aubergine slices for 5 minutes, turning occasionally, until soft and lightly golden.

5 When the quinoa is cooked, drain it and stir in the remaining pomegranate molasses, the pomegranate seeds, cucumber and mint.

6 In a bowl, mix the tahini with the remaining lemon juice.

7 To serve, thinly slice the lamb and serve alongside the pomegranate quinoa and sliced aubergine. Drizzle over the tahini lemon dressing.

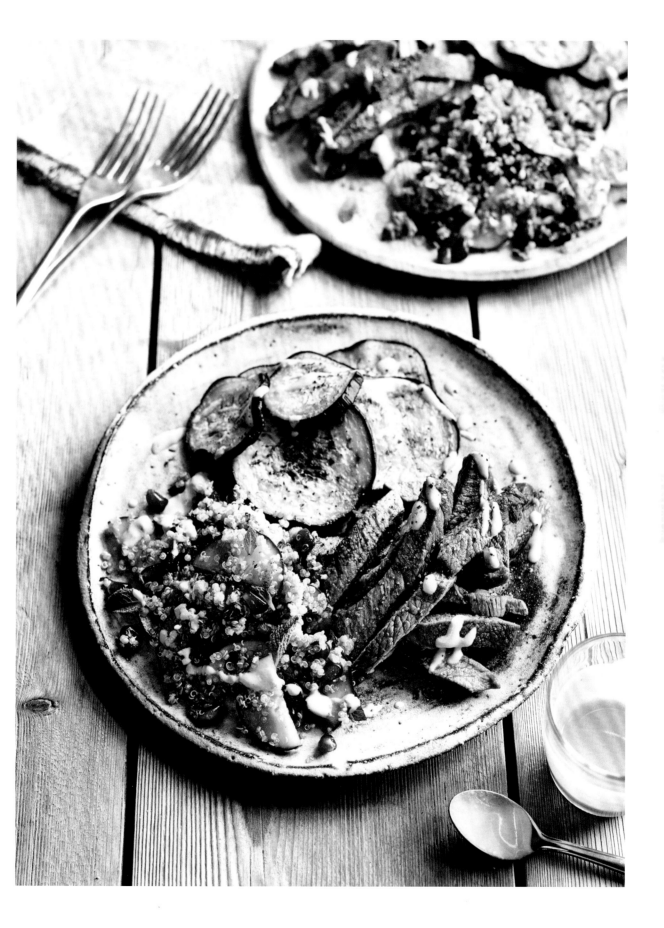

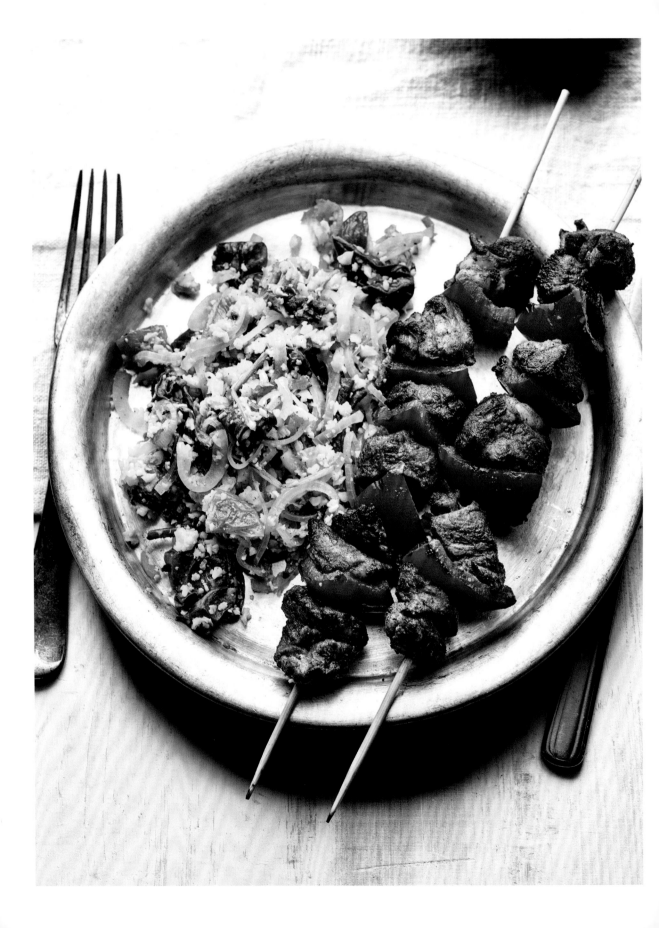

These smoky, chargrilled lamb kebabs are deliciously tender and packed full of flavour, thanks to the warming blend of cumin, chilli, paprika, ginger, cardamom and nutmeg in the the tikka spice. The fragrant cauliflower rice alongside is flavoured with dried apricots for sweetness, crushed cardamom seeds and wonder spice turmeric, which has long been regarded as having a wealth of beneficial properties. Curcumin is the powerful antioxidant in turmeric, giving it its bright golden yellow colour and helping fight free-radical damage.

LAMB TIKKA KEBABS WITH DRIED APRICOTS, CARDAMOM & CAULIFLOWER RICE

1 tbsp tikka spice powder

coconut oil

300g diced lamb shoulder/neck

1 onion

1 red pepper

50g dried apricots

8 cardamom pods

1 cauliflower

½ tsp turmeric

40g spinach

juice of ½ lemon

sea salt and black pepper

4 skewers

1 In a bowl, mix the tikka spice with 1 tablespoon of oil and a pinch of salt. Add the lamb, stir to coat, and set aside to marinate until needed.

2 Finely slice the onion. Cut the red pepper into bite-sized pieces and slice each dried apricot into quarters. Remove the cardamom seeds from the pods, lightly bruise the seeds with a rolling pin or crush in a pestle and mortar, and discard the pods.

3 Using a grater, grate the cauliflower to a rice consistency.

4 Thread pieces of lamb and red pepper alternately on to each skewer.

5 Preheat a griddle pan (or barbecue) on a medium-high heat. Cook the kebabs for 10–15 minutes, turning every 2–3 minutes.

6 Meanwhile, in a medium-sized pan, heat 1 teaspoon of oil on a medium heat and cook the onion, cardamom seeds and turmeric for 5 minutes, until the onion has softened. Add the dried apricots, cauliflower rice and 1 tablespoon of cold water and cook for 3 minutes, stirring frequently.

7 Stir the spinach and lemon juice into the cauliflower rice and cook for 2 minutes, or until the spinach has wilted. Season with salt and pepper.

8 Serve 2 kebabs on each plate, alongside the cauliflower rice.

In the summer, celebrate the season of sweet ripe peaches by making them the star ingredient in this dish. Peaches are a rejuvenating fruit, containing large amounts of antioxidants and vitamin C for healthy skin. We chargrill the fruit, either in a griddle pan or on a barbecue, and serve them with buckwheat, roasted hazelnuts and a zesty lime and chilli dressing.

GRIDDLED PEACHES WITH BUCKWHEAT, TENDERSTEM & HAZELNUTS

½ vegetable stock cube
500ml boiling water
120g buckwheat
1 red onion
200g tenderstem broccoli
30g hazelnuts
olive oil
2 peaches
a handful of fresh mint
½ fresh red chilli
juice of 1 lime
sea salt and black pepper

1 Preheat the oven to 180°C/gas mark 4.

2 Dissolve the vegetable stock cube in the boiling water.

3 Rinse the buckwheat and place in a saucepan with the stock and a pinch of sea salt. Simmer for 15 minutes and then drain.

4 Thinly slice the red onion and trim the tenderstem. Put the onion, tenderstem and hazelnuts on to a baking tray and sprinkle with ½ tablespoon of oil and a pinch of sea salt. Roast in the oven for 10 minutes.

5 Slice each peach into 6 pieces, removing the stone. Drizzle with ½ tablespoon of oil.

6 Heat a griddle pan on a medium-high heat. Add the peaches and cook for 3 minutes each side, until softened and chargrilled.

7 Drain the buckwheat. Finely slice the mint and finely chop the chilli, then stir into the buckwheat along with the roasted onion and tenderstem. Drizzle over half the lime juice, season with black pepper and mix well.

8 Serve the buckwheat on warm plates and top with the griddled peaches. Scatter over the toasted hazelnuts and drizzle over the remaining lime juice.

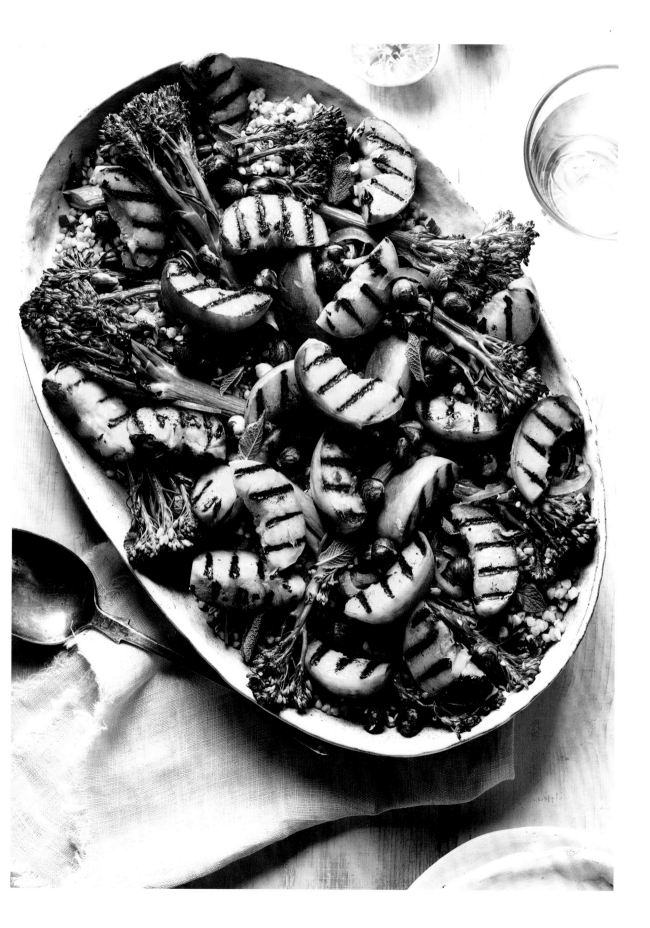

GUT HEALTH

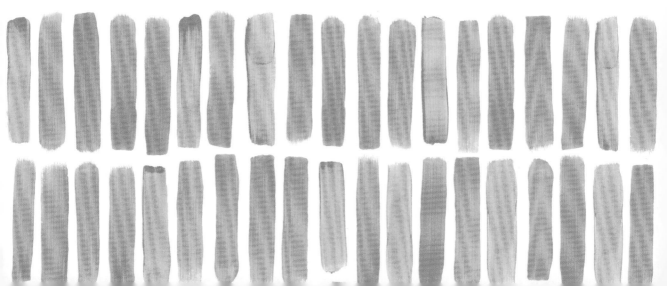

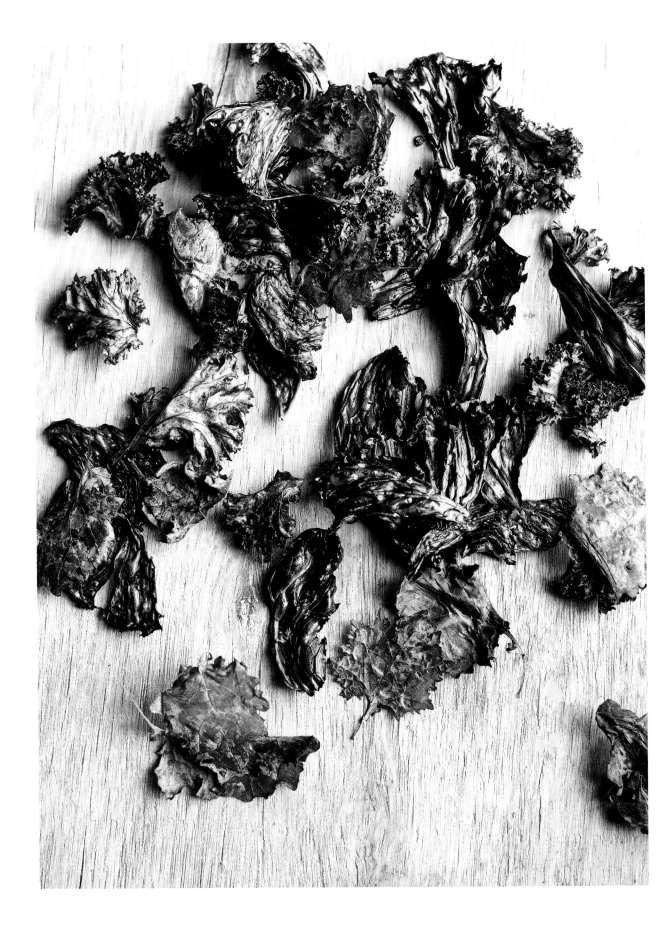

GUT HEALTH

The gut is just as important to us as the brain or the heart. It is one of the most interesting parts of our body, yet most of us know very little about the gut and what it does or how it can affect the way we feel.

More recently, awareness about the gut and its importance to our health has become a hot topic, and you will now hear people refer to it as the body's second brain. The cooperation between the brain and the gut starts at a very early age on a very basic level. Babies vocalise their fundamental needs, such as hunger, by crying. This is a direct relationship between our gut and our brain. But as we grow older we become more reliant upon our sensory organs – eyes, nose and ears. We aren't as focused on the relationship between our gut and our brain because it is harder to quantify than things we can see, smell, touch or hear. However, that relationship doesn't just go away, it becomes more complex and is the reason we feel a lot of the emotions we do.

WHAT DOES THE GUT DO AND HOW CAN IT CHANGE THE WAY WE FEEL?

Research has shown that digestive problems in the gut can negatively influence the way we feel. When the gut is stressed it sends signals to the part of the brain that produces negative feelings. If this is true, then can fixing our gut really change the way we feel? Could it be the case that if we are eating well and our gut is healthy we will in turn feel a lot better within ourselves? I believe so, and I am going to explain how you can do this.

The gut is the largest immune system organ we have and it communicates with all the cells in our body. Its job is to allow nutrients and water to enter the body while preventing toxins from passing through. This will only happen, however, if the gut is healthy. If its health becomes compromised, it will allow toxins to enter and that's when problems start to occur.

Your gut should have a good balance of bacteria and a healthy gut lining and immune system. To maintain all three is relatively easy to do through good nutrition. It is when you start making poor food choices or if you are intolerant to certain foods that one of the three will be compromised and will cause you problems. Take the gut lining, for example. When the gut wall becomes irritated the lining becomes more permeable and allows bad bacteria through. This is known as leaky gut syndrome and is fairly common. It can be caused by excessive sugar, refined carbohydrates, excessive alcohol consumption, parasites or stress, among other things. Why is it so common? Well, a lot of the food we eat today wasn't around 100 years ago and our gut struggles to process it. This is evident in the ever-increasing number of people suffering from some sort of food intolerance, and it is one of the reasons Mindful Chef promotes eating whole, natural, unprocessed foods – in other words – getting back to basics.

I am lucky that I have not suffered from any serious conditions such as IBS, but I have suffered food intolerances on a very ad hoc basis. During my time at university, right up until about two years ago (when I became really interested in nutrition and started researching more), I would suffer the most debilitating stomach cramps. They would have me rolled up into a ball on the floor, as it felt as though my stomach was being ripped from my body. These episodes were not only extremely painful but I would sweat a lot and feel very sick. I knew it must be something I was eating, but as they happened on such a rare basis I didn't pay too much attention to them and carried on my daily routine, despite occasionally having moments that brought my life to a standstill for the best part of an hour.

Two years ago, having read more about the gut and its relationship with the body, I finally decided to take matters into my own hands and do something about these cramps by speaking to a nutritional therapist. After eliminating foods from my diet and reintroducing them gradually, I was able to figure out exactly what types of food were causing me these problems and as a result I haven't had any episodes since. I cannot tell you how great it was to know that there was something that could be done. It felt as though a massive weight was lifted and I was finally going to get rid of these problems once and for all. Today I also feel a lot better knowing I am eating the right types of food for my body; in turn I feel more positive and energetic than ever before.

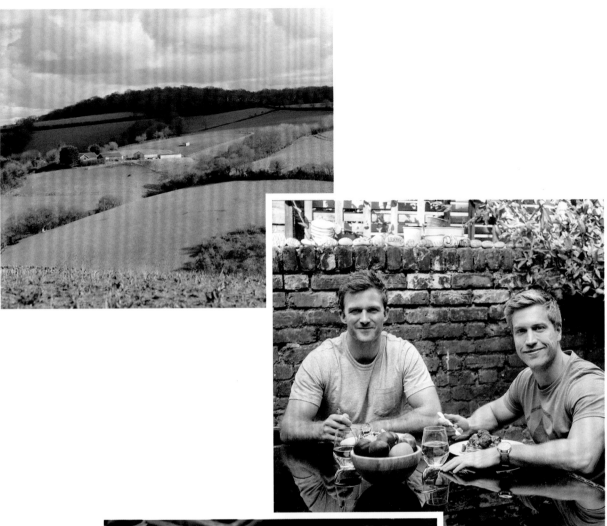

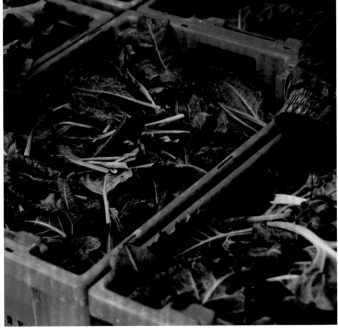

At Mindful Chef we know that not everyone suffers from gluten sensitivity but we believe reducing the amount of it in your diet will be beneficial for most people

WHAT CAUSES GUT PROBLEMS?

For the most part it is the foods we eat. Although remember that we are all different, so what may be problematic for me may, in fact, be absolutely fine for you. Some of the most common foods that cause the gut problems are gluten, lactose (dairy), fructose (fruit sugars) and lectins (a type of protein found in grains, legumes and some dairy products). In less serious cases most people simply don't have the ability to be able to process these foods. One in a hundred people suffer from coeliac disease, but a much higher percentage of the population will suffer from gluten sensitivity – anything from bloating, to mild feelings of discomfort, to headaches and flatulence. It is when people start to reduce the amount of gluten in their diet that they limit the amount of stress placed on the gut and start to see an improvement in their general wellbeing. At Mindful Chef we know that not everyone suffers from gluten sensitivity but we believe reducing the amount of it in your diet will be beneficial for most people. That is one of the reasons we choose to keep our recipes gluten-free.

HOW CAN YOU KEEP YOUR GUT HEALTHY?

Fibre is essential for maintaining a healthy gut and you can find it in abundance in vegetables, fruits and grains. Essentially fibre performs two vital functions: it helps food move through the digestive system, removing toxins, and it can fuel the good bacteria found in the large intestine. There are two forms of fibre – insoluble and soluble. Insoluble fibre cannot be digested easily but helps move food through the digestive system. Seeds, nuts and leafy greens are good examples of insoluble fibre. Soluble fibre, which is found in foods like oats, bananas and oranges, dissolves in water in the gut and helps make stools softer, making them easier to pass through your body.

TOP 5 WAYS YOU CAN HELP KEEP YOUR GUT HEALTHY EVERY DAY

1. **EAT REAL, 'WHOLE' FOODS**

   Thousands of years ago people didn't suffer from the same problems we do now, and that has to be in some part due to the advancements in food technology and manufacturing. The body finds it harder to digest processed foods full of preservatives and additives. Get back to basics and eat whole food and real sources of proteins, carbohydrates and fats.

2. **EAT MORE FIBRE**

   We can all be guilty of not eating enough vegetables and fruit. Ideally we should be eating vegetables at every meal, but many of us are only including them in our evening meals. Low carbohydrate diets are guilty of reducing the amount of good bacteria in our gut (remember, fibre fuels good bacteria and is present in a lot of carbohydrates), which is why we don't promote a particular diet but more of a balanced, well-rounded approach.

3. **MANAGE YOUR STRESS AND SLEEP WELL**

   This point is so important that we have dedicated two chapters in our book to it. We perform vital functions when sleeping and perform them better when we aren't stressed. This can help with inflammation and in turn may improve gut health.

4. **CREATE A HEALTHY BALANCE OF BACTERIA IN YOUR GUT**

   Having more good bacteria will strengthen the intestinal barrier and create a healthy environment for the body to thrive. Good bacteria helps to make vitamins, fight pathogens and digest food. Eating enough fibre is important for gut health and regulates pH balance in the gut, helping the good bacteria to flourish.

5. **FIND OUT WHAT'S CAUSING THE PROBLEM**

   For me it was a combination of certain foods taken at a certain time. The problem was exacerbated by eating them just before exercise. Having removed the foods and reintroduced them at a different time of the day, I have not experienced the same cramps since.

All the recipes in this chapter have been picked because we believe that when combined with a healthy diet, they can improve your overall gut health and digestion. The ingredients in these meals are all made from real food and are high in fibre.

We've created our own delicious vegan version of the traditional Vietnamese noodle soup 'pho' and have infused it with aromatic star anise and packed it with a range of nutrient-rich vegetables. We've added tofu stir-fried in tamari, plus a sprinkling of cashew nuts for protein.

VIETNAMESE PHO WITH COURGETTE NOODLES, TOFU & CASHEWS

1 vegetable stock cube
500ml boiling water
2 garlic cloves
1 fresh red chilli
100g tenderstem broccoli
100g oyster mushrooms
1 red pepper
300g firm tofu
300g courgettes
coconut oil
2 tsp tamari
2 star anise
50g cashew nuts

1 Dissolve the stock cube in the boiling water and set aside.

2 Finely chop the garlic and finely slice the chilli (remove the seeds for less heat). Chop the tenderstem into 2.5cm pieces and halve the mushrooms lengthways. Thinly slice the red pepper. Drain and rinse the tofu, cut it into 2cm cubes and pat dry with kitchen paper.

3 Remove the ends of the courgettes, but leave the skin on. Peel the courgette into ribbons then slice the ribbons lengthways into long thin strands (or use a julienne peeler or spiraliser, if you have one, to make noodles).

4 Heat ½ tablespoon of oil in a frying pan, then add the tofu and half the garlic and fry for 5 minutes. Add the tamari and fry for a further 5 minutes, until the tofu is golden brown.

5 Meanwhile, heat ½ tablespoon of oil in a medium-sized pan and fry the remaining garlic for a minute, then add the mushrooms, tenderstem, red pepper and star anise and cook for 3 minutes.

6 Add the vegetable stock and courgette noodles to this pan and simmer for 5 minutes. Turn off the heat and carefully remove the star anise.

7 Serve the vegetable soup in bowls, topped with the tofu and sprinkled with the sliced chilli and cashew nuts. Enjoy!

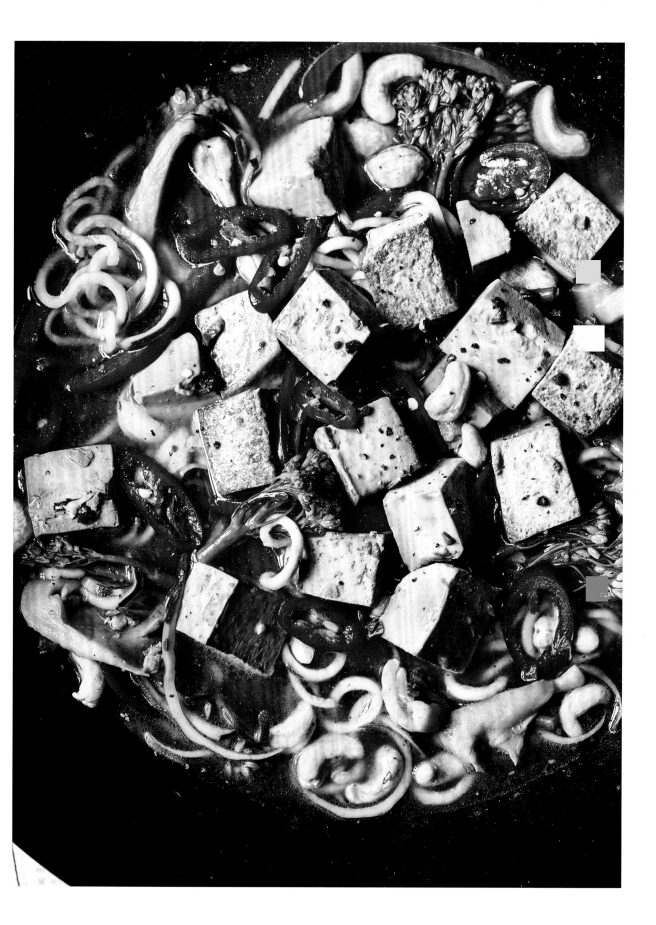

Inspired by the fragrant flavours of the southern Indian state of Kerala, this delicate fish curry is made with garlic, ginger and crushed cardamom seeds, great for improving digestion. We use monkfish as it holds its shape well, but you could use any firm white fish. Quick and comforting, this beats a takeaway any night of the week.

KERALAN COCONUT & MONKFISH CURRY WITH CORIANDER & WILD RICE

80g wild rice
400ml boiling water
2 garlic cloves
1 fresh green chilli
4cm fresh ginger
6 cardamom pods
1 red onion
4 tomatoes
300g monkfish
coconut oil
1 tsp turmeric
200ml coconut milk
handful of fresh coriander
sea salt and black pepper

1 Rinse the wild rice and put into a saucepan with the boiling water. Cook on a medium heat for 25–30 minutes, then add a pinch of salt.

2 Meanwhile, finely chop the garlic and chilli and peel and finely chop the ginger. Remove the cardamom seeds from the pods, lightly bruise the seeds with a rolling pin or crush with a pestle and mortar, and discard the pods. Finely slice the red onion and slice the tomatoes. Cut the monkfish into bite-sized pieces.

3 Heat 1 teaspoon of oil in a pan and add the garlic, ginger, chilli and cardamom seeds and cook for 1 minute. Add the red onion and fry for 5 minutes, until softened.

4 Add the turmeric and monkfish pieces to the pan, stirring to coat the fish with the turmeric. Add the coconut milk, season with sea salt and black pepper and simmer for 5 minutes to reduce the sauce slightly, stirring occasionally.

5 Add the sliced tomatoes and cook for a further 5 minutes, until the fish is cooked through.

6 Roughly chop half the coriander leaves and stir into the curry. Drain the wild rice.

7 Serve the wild rice in bowls and top with the monkfish curry. Garnish with the remaining coriander.

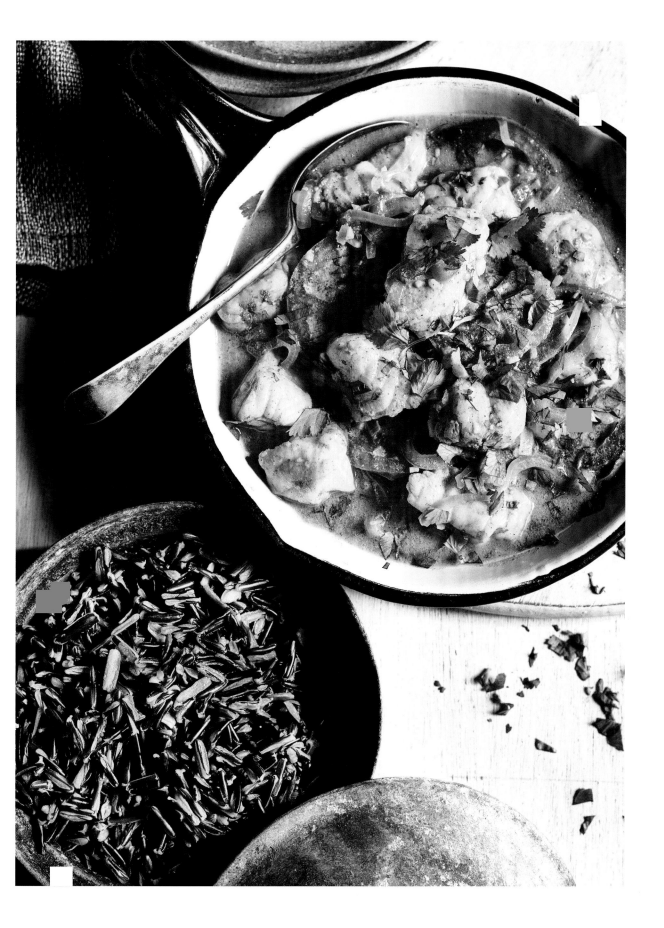

These spinach and chickpea falafels are served with a refreshing kale, avocado and pomegranate salad. The kale is drizzled with tangy apple cider vinegar, to help detoxify the body. If you have time, it's worth massaging the dressing into the kale for a minute or two with your hands to soften the leaves and allow them to really take on the surrounding flavours. Removing pomegranate seeds can be quite a messy experience – to make this easier and quicker, slice the pomegranate in half, hold over a bowl and tap the back firmly with a wooden spoon to release the seeds.

SPINACH FALAFELS WITH COCONUT HARISSA SAUCE & ZINGY KALE SALAD

240g drained chickpeas
100g spinach
2 tbsp chickpea flour
olive oil
80g kale
½ pomegranate
1 avocado
20g walnuts
1½ tbsp apple cider vinegar
15g creamed coconut
2 tbsp boiling water
1 tsp harissa paste
sea salt and black pepper

1 Preheat the oven to 200°C/gas mark 6.

2 Put the chickpeas into a bowl and mash for 1–2 minutes with a potato masher or the back of a fork, until they are all crushed.

3 Place the spinach in a separate bowl. Pour over enough boiling water to cover and leave to wilt for 1 minute. Place the spinach in a sieve and drain off the excess water, then finely chop.

4 Add the spinach to the chickpeas. Add the chickpea flour, 1 teaspoon of olive oil and 1 tablespoon of water, season generously and mix well. Form the chickpea mixture into 12 balls, place them on a baking tray, and bake in the oven for 15–20 minutes, turning them halfway through.

5 Meanwhile, make the kale salad. Finely slice the kale (removing any tough stalks). Cut the pomegranate in half and remove the seeds. Peel and de-stone the avocado and cut it into small pieces. Roughly chop the walnuts. Put the kale into a bowl and mix in the apple cider vinegar and ½ tablespoon of oil. Add the pomegranate seeds, avocado and walnuts and season with salt and pepper.

6 Dissolve the creamed coconut in the boiling water and mix with the harissa paste.

7 Serve the falafels on plates and drizzle over the coconut harissa sauce. Serve alongside the zingy kale salad.

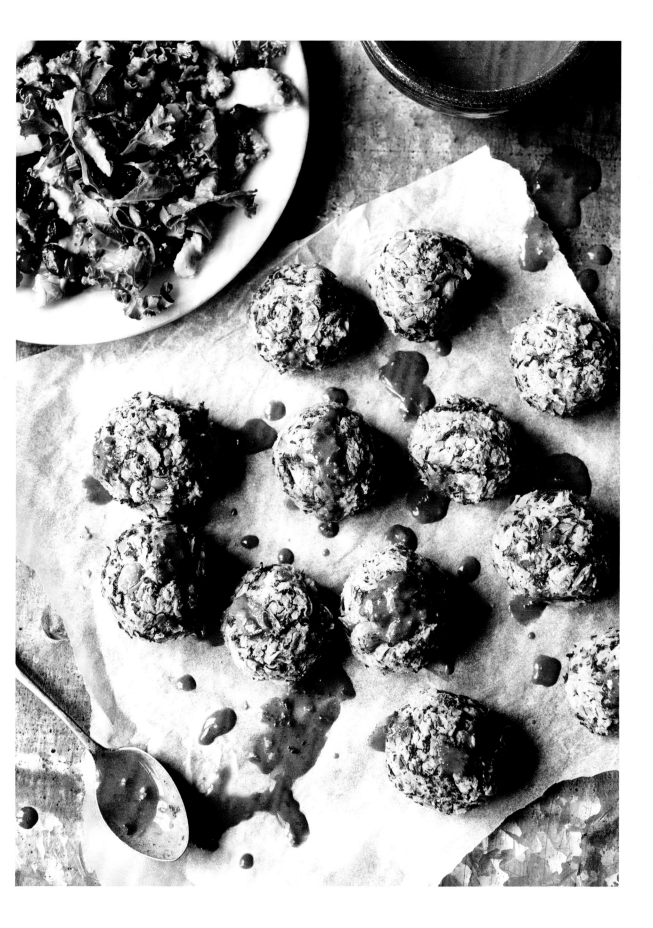

This comforting dish is so hearty and satisfying that you won't miss the meat. The chestnuts and mushrooms add an earthy flavour that is delicious with the tangy richness of the sun-dried tomatoes and the sweet potato and thyme mash. We used pre-cooked chestnuts to save on time, but you could roast fresh chestnuts if you have some available. Chestnuts are in season from late autumn through the winter, and compared to other nuts are low in fat, plus they have lots of dietary fibre, which is important for digestive health.

VEGAN 'SHEPHERD'S PIE' WITH SWEET POTATO, CHESTNUTS & MUSHROOMS

2 garlic cloves
160g mushrooms
80g kale
40g pre-cooked chestnuts
40g sun-dried tomatoes
olive oil
1 vegetable stock cube
100ml boiling water
240g drained butter beans
2 sprigs of fresh thyme
200g passata
300g sweet potatoes
sea salt and black pepper

1 Finely chop or crush the garlic and finely slice the mushrooms. Roughly chop the kale, chestnuts and sun-dried tomatoes.

2 Heat ½ tablespoon of oil in a medium-sized pan. Add the garlic, mushrooms and kale and cook for 5 minutes, until softened.

3 Dissolve the stock cube in the boiling water.

4 Add the drained butter beans and the stock to the same pan as the vegetables, along with the chestnuts, sun-dried tomatoes, the leaves from a sprig of thyme and the passata. Mix well and leave to simmer for 15 minutes, until the sauce has thickened.

5 Meanwhile, peel the sweet potatoes and chop into 1cm cubes. Place in a pan of boiling water with a pinch of sea salt and boil for 10 minutes, until soft.

6 Preheat the grill to high. Drain the sweet potatoes, then mash with a potato masher or the back of a fork. Stir in the leaves from a sprig of thyme.

7 Place the vegetable and bean mix in a small ovenproof dish and top with the sweet potato mash. Grill for 5 minutes, until golden brown.

This vegetarian take on a Bolognese sauce replaces the meat with brown lentils for a satisfying texture. Including lentils in your diet is great for your digestive health, and the fibre can even help regulate cholesterol levels. If you'd rather not wait for the dried lentils to cook, you could use ready-to-eat lentils from a packet or tin – just give them a good rinse and add them for the last 5–10 minutes of the cooking time – enough to heat them.

RICH LENTIL & TOMATO BOLOGNESE WITH COURGETTI & PINE NUTS

80g dried brown lentils
300ml boiling water
2 garlic cloves
120g carrots
120g chestnut mushrooms
180g cherry tomatoes
4 sprigs of fresh thyme
olive oil
200g passata
2 tbsp sun-dried tomato paste
300g courgettes
30g pine nuts
sea salt and black pepper

1 Rinse the lentils and place them in a pan with the boiling water and a pinch of salt. Simmer for 25–30 minutes, until tender.

2 Meanwhile, finely chop the garlic. Peel and finely dice the carrots. Finely slice the mushrooms and cut the tomatoes in half. Remove the leaves from the thyme sprigs.

3 Heat 1 teaspoon of oil in a large pan, add the garlic and carrots, and cook for 5 minutes. Add the mushrooms and tomatoes and cook for 5 minutes more, until all the vegetables have softened.

4 Add the passata, sun-dried tomato paste and thyme leaves and cook for a further 5 minutes. Season with salt and pepper.

5 Meanwhile, remove the ends of the courgettes, but leave the skin on. Prepare the courgetti by peeling the courgette into ribbons then slice the ribbons lengthways into long thin strands (or use a julienne peeler or spiraliser, if you have one, to make noodles).

6 Heat 1 teaspoon of oil in another pan. Add the courgetti and cook for 2 minutes, until the courgetti begin to soften.

7 Drain the lentils and stir into the vegetables. To serve, place the courgette noodles on plates and spoon over the lentil bolognese. Scatter over the pine nuts.

Seaweed is a remarkable superfood, containing fibre, protein and an impressive range of minerals – such as iodine, needed for thyroid function, calcium for building and maintaining strong bones, iron for transporting oxygen around the body, and magnesium for a healthy immune system. Seaweed is definitely a food group we should be eating much more of. Look for sustainably sourced, hand-harvested seaweed if possible, to support the local ecosystem.

BAKED SALMON WITH CRISPY SEAWEED, POACHED EGG & ASPARAGUS

400ml boiling water
80g millet
1 lemon
140g asparagus
2 x 150g salmon fillets
olive oil
2 eggs
60g spinach
2 dried nori sheets
sea salt and black pepper

1 Preheat the oven to 180°C/gas mark 4.

2 Heat a saucepan, then pour in the millet and toast it for 2 minutes, stirring constantly. Pour in the boiling water, reduce the heat, then cover the pan and cook for 15 minutes.

3 Thinly slice half the lemon and cut the slices into half-moons. Trim the asparagus.

4 Place the salmon fillets on a baking tray, layer over the lemon slices and drizzle 1 teaspoon of oil over each fillet. Place the asparagus alongside, drizzle with 1 teaspoon of oil and season with black pepper. Place the salmon in the oven for 12–15 minutes, or until cooked to your liking.

5 Bring another saucepan of water to a gentle simmer. Create a whirlpool in the pan with a spoon, then carefully break the eggs into the middle, one at a time. Cook for 3–4 minutes, until the whites are cooked, then remove from the pan.

6 Once the millet is cooked, stir in the spinach for 2–3 minutes, until wilted, then drain and stir in the juice of the remaining lemon half. Break up the nori sheets and place on a serving plate.

7 Spoon the spinach millet on to plates, place a salmon fillet on top, and sprinkle over the nori, crumbling it if you want smaller pieces. Serve with the asparagus, topped with the poached egg and a sprinkle of salt.

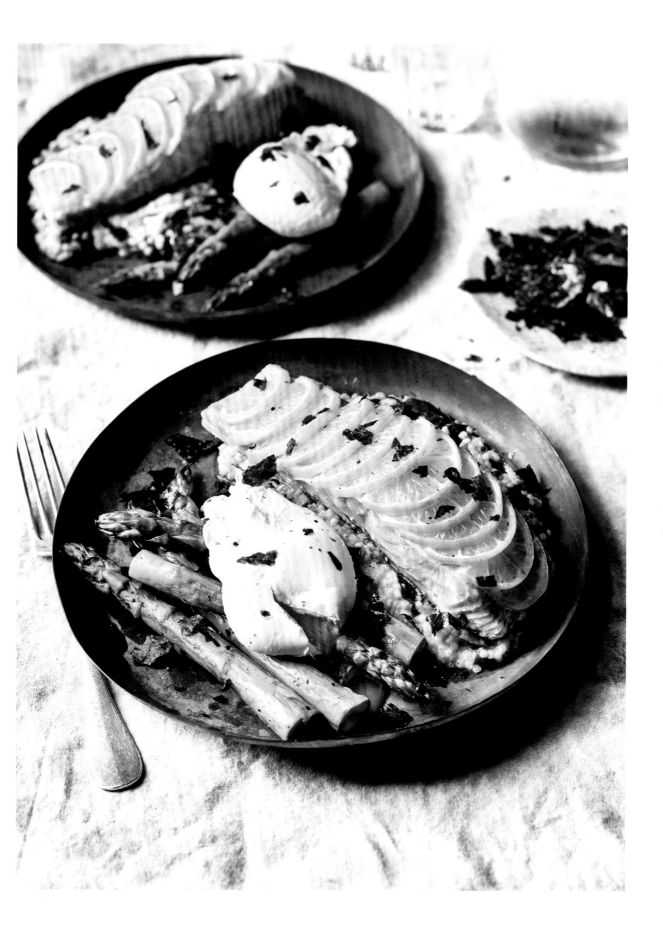

This aromatic Moroccan inspired tagine has a rich flavour from the ras el hanout, an aromatic mix of spices including paprika, coriander, cumin, cardamom and rose petals. We've added preserved lemons for a zingy finish – the lemons are preserved in a brine solution which makes the peel soft and tangy. Cauliflower helps the liver detoxify the body, and is a great source of vitamin C for protecting against colds and flu.

CHICKEN THIGH & PRESERVED LEMON TAGINE WITH CAULIFLOWER RICE

1 onion
2 garlic cloves
olive oil
4 chicken thighs, skinless
    and boneless
40g preserved lemons
80g green beans
½ chicken stock cube
300ml boiling water
1 tbsp ras el hanout
60g pitted black olives
20g flaked almonds
1 cauliflower
sea salt and black pepper

1 Finely slice the onion and finely chop the garlic.

2 Heat ½ tablespoon of oil in a medium-sized pan on a medium heat and fry the onion and garlic for 2 minutes. Season the chicken thighs and add to the pan, then fry for 5 minutes each side.

3 Slice the preserved lemons into quarters. Trim the green beans and slice in half. Dissolve the stock cube in the boiling water.

4 Add the ras el hanout to the chicken, then add the stock, preserved lemons and black olives. Simmer with a lid on for a further 10 minutes, then add the green beans and simmer with the lid off for 5 minutes, or until the chicken is cooked through and the beans are tender.

5 Meanwhile, heat a dry frying pan on a medium-high heat and toast the flaked almonds for 3 minutes, until turning golden brown. Remove from the pan.

6 Grate the cauliflower to a rice consistency using a grater. Using the same frying pan, heat 1 teaspoon of oil over a gentle heat. Add the cauliflower rice and cook for 3–4 minutes, stirring constantly, until it has softened slightly.

7 Season with salt and pepper, then take off the heat and stir in the toasted almonds. Spoon the chicken tagine into warm bowls, and serve with the cauliflower rice.

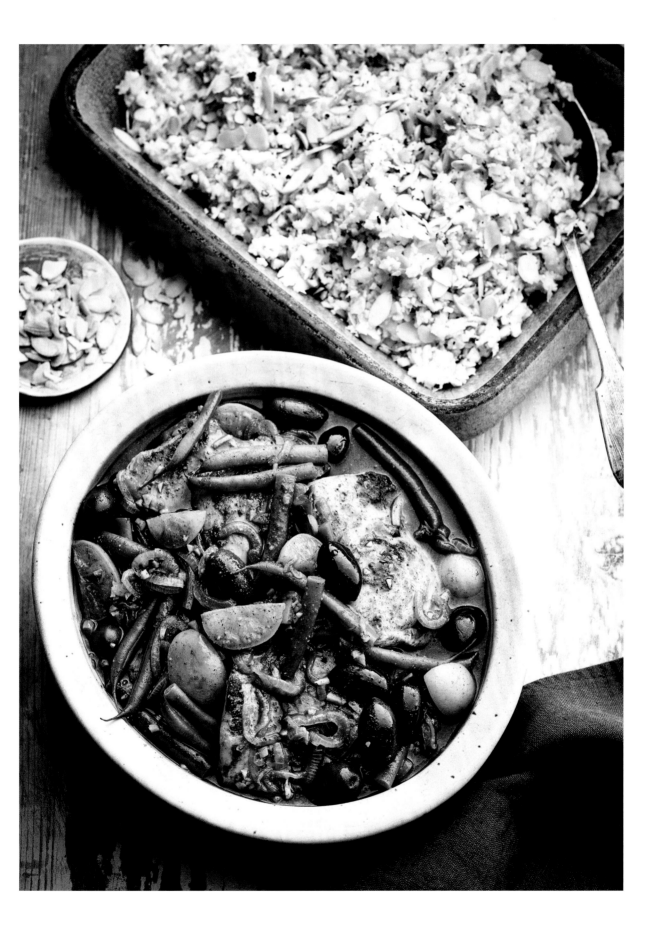

This is a super-speedy and comforting roast for those days where you don't have more than 30 minutes to spare! Parsnips are a great partner to lamb, but instead of roasting them we've boiled and mashed these for a tasty and lighter alternative to starchy white potatoes. Purple carrots are a vibrant accompaniment, and contain antioxidants lutein and lycopene for eye health. The purple variety contains even more antioxidant pigments than orange carrots. The simple homemade mint sauce is bursting with fresh mint to aid digestion.

LAMB STEAK WITH HOMEMADE MINT SAUCE, PARSNIP MASH & ROASTED PURPLE CARROTS

400g parsnips
160g green beans
200g purple carrots
1 red onion
olive oil
a handful of fresh thyme
2 x 150g lamb leg steaks
handful of fresh mint
2 tbsp white wine vinegar
2 tsp honey
sea salt and black pepper

1 Preheat the oven to 200°C/gas mark 6.

2 Peel the parsnips and chop into 1cm cubes and trim the green beans. Peel the carrots and slice into batons. Cut the red onion into chunks.

3 Place the carrot and onion on a baking tray, drizzle over ½ tablespoon of oil and sprinkle over the leaves from the thyme and a pinch of sea salt. Roast in the oven for 20–25 minutes.

4 Season the lamb steaks. Heat ½ tablespoon of oil in a frying pan on a medium-high heat and brown the lamb for 2 minutes each side.

5 Place the lamb on a baking tray and roast it for 10–15 minutes for medium–rare; longer for well done. Leave to rest for a few minutes.

6 Meanwhile, place the parsnips in a saucepan of boiling water and simmer for 10 minutes, then add the beans to the pan and cook for a further 4 minutes, until tender. Drain the vegetables and set aside the beans. Mash the parsnips with a potato masher and cover to keep warm.

7 To make the mint sauce, finely chop the mint leaves. Mix the vinegar and honey together in a bowl until the honey dissolves. Then stir in the chopped mint and season to taste.

8 Spoon the mash on to warm plates and top with the lamb. Drizzle over the mint sauce and serve with the carrots, onion and green beans.

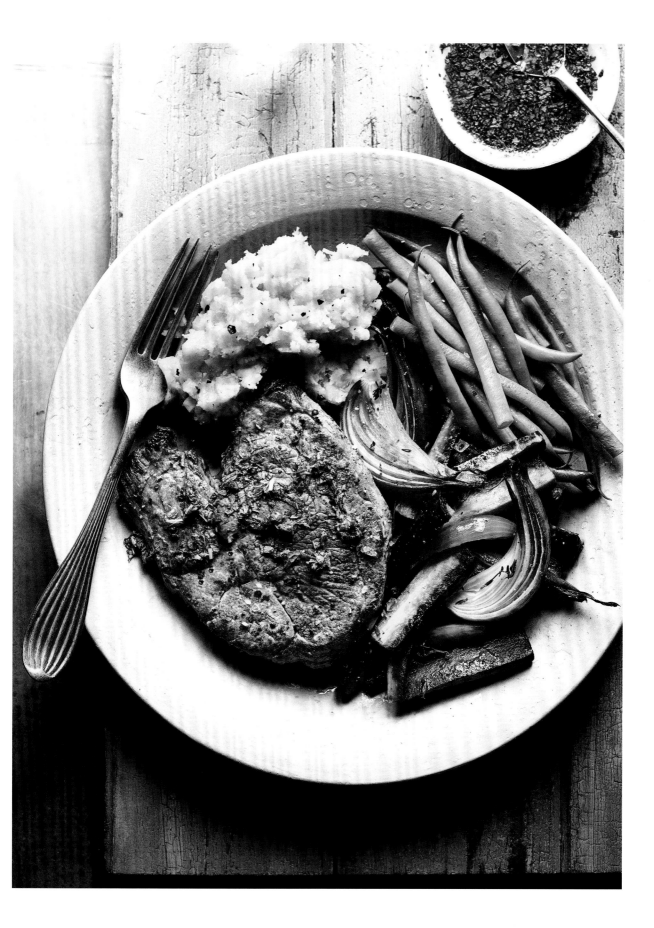

This is such an easy mid-week supper, as the vegetables are roasted in the oven along with the juicy chicken thighs. We opt for boneless chicken thighs as they cook quicker, and skinless to reduce the amount of fat in the dish. We coat the chicken in a sweet, sticky sauce of honey and tamari with fragrant crushed cardamom seeds, which are great for improving digestion. The quinoa soaks up the delicious juices from the chicken, but if you prefer brown rice this would work equally well.

CARDAMOM & HONEY CHICKEN THIGHS WITH GREEN BEANS & QUINOA

1 red pepper
140g green beans
2 garlic cloves
8 cardamom pods
4 chicken thighs, skinless and
    boneless
1 tbsp honey
2 tbsp tamari
olive oil
80g quinoa
300ml boiling water
20g flaked almonds
sea salt and black pepper

1 Preheat the oven to 200°C/gas mark 6.

2 Chop the red pepper into bite-sized pieces and trim the green beans. Finely chop or crush the garlic. Remove the cardamom seeds from the pods, lightly bruise the seeds with a rolling pin or crush with a pestle and mortar and discard the pods. Slice each chicken thigh in half.

3 To make the cardamom and honey sauce, mix the honey, tamari, garlic and cardamom seeds in a bowl with 1 tablespoon of olive oil and season with black pepper. Add the chicken to the bowl and stir to coat.

4 Place the chicken and sauce in an ovenproof dish with the red pepper and place in the oven for 20 minutes, until the chicken is golden brown and cooked through.

5 Rinse the quinoa and place in a pan with the boiling water and a pinch of sea salt. Simmer for 15 minutes, then drain. Place the green beans in a steamer, cover and steam for 4–5 minutes, until tender, then set aside and keep warm.

6 When the chicken thighs are cooked, remove them from the oven. Mix the red pepper and the juices from the pan with the quinoa.

7 To serve, spoon the quinoa and peppers on to warm plates. Layer over the green beans, followed by the chicken thighs then sprinkle over the flaked almonds.

This summery Vietnamese-style crispy pork is bursting with flavour and is served on a bed of bright and nourishing red pepper, courgetti and carrot noodles. The pork is sprinkled with crunchy peanuts, fresh lime and chopped fresh mint, a soothing herb for promoting digestion.

VIETNAMESE CRISPY PORK WITH COURGETTE & CARROT NOODLES

2 tbsp tamari
1 tbsp fish sauce
2 tsp honey
juice of 2 limes
4cm fresh ginger
coconut oil
300g pork mince
200g carrots
300g courgettes
1 red pepper
handful of fresh mint leaves
20g peanuts
black pepper

1 To make the sauce, mix the tamari, fish sauce, honey, and half the lime juice in a bowl.

2 Peel and finely chop or grate the ginger. Heat ½ tablespoon of oil in a wok or frying pan on a medium-high heat. Add the ginger and cook for 1 minute, then add the pork mince, breaking it up with a spoon, and cook for 10 minutes. Add half the sauce and cook for a further 10 minutes, until the pork begins to turn crispy.

3 While the pork is cooking, make the carrot and courgette noodles. Peel the carrots, then prepare the noodles using a spiraliser or julienne peeler (or if you don't have one, use a peeler to slice the carrot into long thin strips). Repeat with the courgettes, leaving the skin on, but removing
the ends.

4 Thinly slice the red pepper, finely chop the mint and roughly chop or crush the peanuts.

5 Heat 1 teaspoon of oil in a medium-sized pan. Add the carrot and courgette noodles, along with the red pepper and the remaining sauce, and cook for 3–5 minutes, until the vegetables have softened slightly. Stir in half the mint and season with pepper.

6 Transfer the noodles and red pepper to warm plates, and spoon over the pork mince. Sprinkle over the peanuts and the rest of the mint and drizzle over the remaining lime juice.

A peeler makes it possible to create ribbons or noodles out of almost every root vegetable – we urge you to give it a go! The mineral-packed sweet parsnip ribbons are baked in the oven until they turn crispy, then topped with the meatballs and drizzled with an Italian-inspired gremolata. The gremolata is packed with lemon zest, garlic and parsley, and we've added chopped hazelnuts for their nutrients– it's a great immunity-boosting dish.

PORK & LEMON MEATBALLS WITH PARSNIP RIBBONS & HAZELNUT GREMOLATA

2 garlic cloves
handful of fresh flat-leaf parsley
handful of cherry tomatoes
1 aubergine
20g hazelnuts
400g parsnips
olive oil
300g pork mince
zest and juice of 1 lemon
60g spinach
sea salt and black pepper

1 Preheat the oven to 180°C/gas mark 4.

2 Finely chop the garlic and parsley. Slice the cherry tomatoes in half and cut the aubergine into 2cm cubes. Roughly chop the hazelnuts.

3 Peel the parsnips, then, using a peeler, make long thin strips and place on a baking tray. Toss with 2 teaspoons of oil and sprinkle with a pinch of sea salt. Bake in the oven for 10–15 minutes, until beginning to crisp around the edges.

4 Meanwhile, in a bowl, mix together the pork mince, half the garlic, half the lemon zest, half the lemon juice and half the parsley. Form the mixture into 12 meatballs.

5 Heat 1 teaspoon of oil in a frying pan on a medium-high heat and fry the meatballs on all sides for 10–15 minutes, until golden and cooked through.

6 Meanwhile, in a separate pan, heat 1 teaspoon of oil on a medium heat. Add the aubergine and fry for 5 minutes, then add the tomatoes and spinach for another 5 minutes. Season with salt and pepper.

7 To make the gremolata, mix together the remaining garlic, parsley lemon zest and juice in a bowl and add the chopped hazelnuts. Season.

8 To serve, place the parsnip ribbons on warm plates, spoon over the aubergine, tomatoes and spinach and top with the meatballs. Drizzle over the hazelnut gremolata.

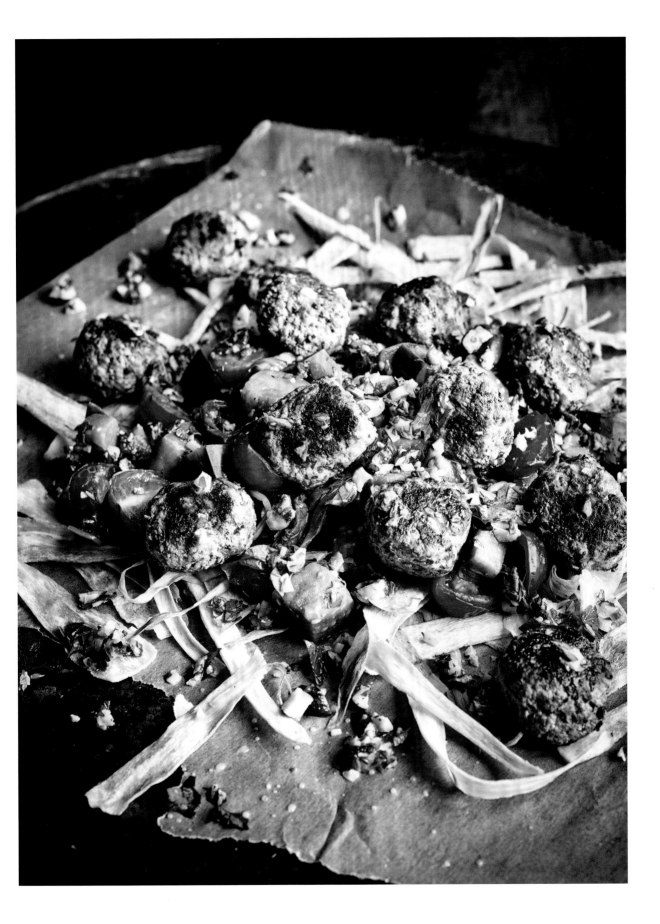

We've roasted succulent organic lamb steak with fragrant rosemary and served them on a bed of cannellini beans and sun-dried tomatoes. Rosemary is a fragrant herb that pairs beautifully with lamb and stimulates cognitive ability by improving circulation. We've also added crunchy kale crisps, rich in calcium to keep bones strong. Kale crisps make a nutritious snack for any time of the day – just sprinkle over your preferred spice with a drizzle of coconut oil or olive oil and bake.

ROSEMARY LAMB WITH ITALIAN CANNELLINI BEANS & KALE CRISPS

2 garlic cloves
1 red onion
3 sprigs of fresh rosemary
150g cherry tomatoes
60g kale
40g sun-dried tomatoes
olive oil
2 x 150g lamb leg steaks
240g drained cannellini beans
1 tbsp balsamic vinegar
sea salt and black pepper

1 Preheat the oven to 200°C/gas mark 6.

2 Finely chop or crush the garlic and finely slice the red onion. Finely chop the rosemary, removing the stalks. Slice the cherry tomatoes in half. Roughly chop the kale leaves, removing the tough stalks, and roughly chop the sun-dried tomatoes.

3 Heat ½ tablespoon of oil in a frying pan on a medium heat. Season the lamb steaks and cook for 2–3 minutes on each side, then remove from the pan and place on a baking tray. Sprinkle over half the rosemary and 1 teaspoon of oil and place in the oven for 10–15 minutes, until cooked but still slightly pink in the middle. Leave to rest for 5 minutes.

4 Meanwhile, heat ½ tablespoon of oil in a medium-sized pan on a medium heat. Add the garlic and the remaining rosemary and cook for 1 minute, then add the red onion and cook for a further 7 minutes, until softened and turning golden.

5 Drain the beans and add to the red onion, along with the sun-dried tomatoes, balsamic vinegar, cherry tomatoes and 2 tablespoons of water. Simmer for 5–10 minutes, then season.

6 While the lamb is resting, place the kale on a baking tray, drizzle over 1 teaspoon of oil and place in the oven for 5 minutes, until crispy.

7 Thinly slice the lamb steaks. To serve, spoon the Italian beans on to warm plates, sprinkle over the kale crisps and place the sliced lamb on top.

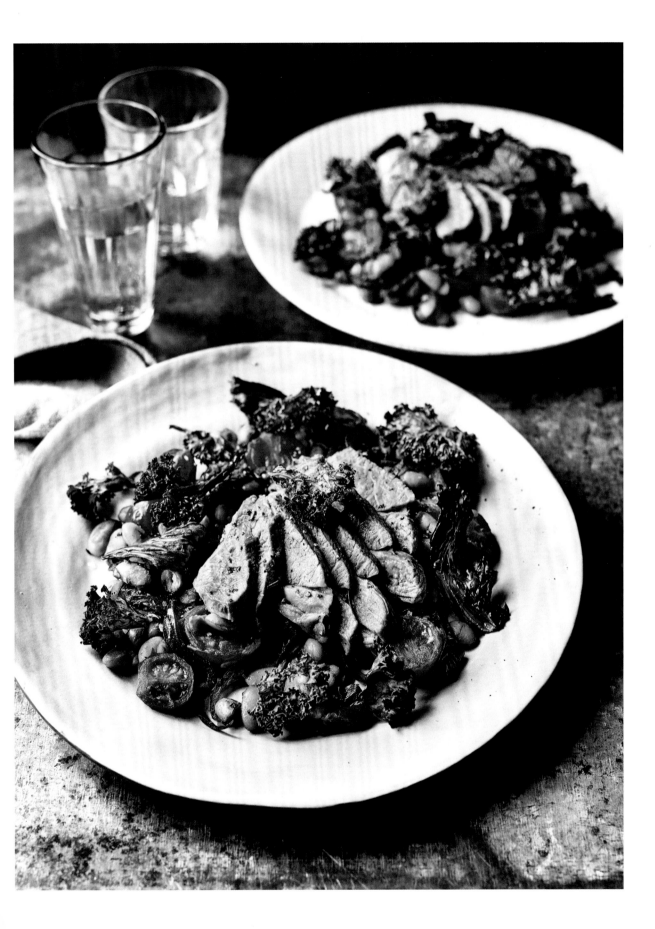

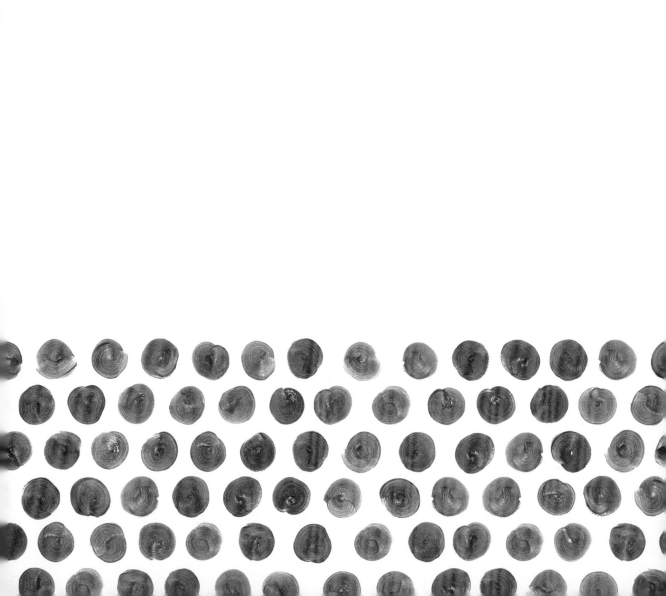

EXERCISE

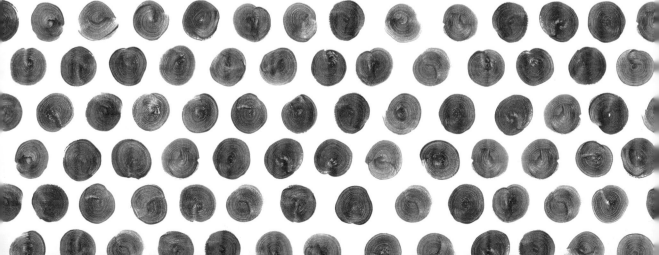

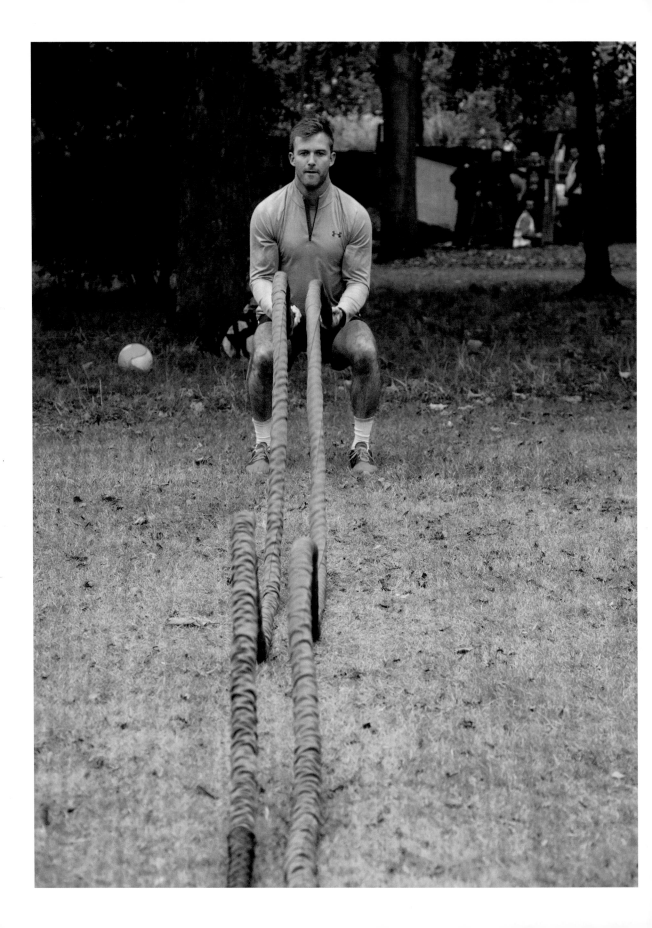

EXERCISE

Our bodies are amazing things and are capable of doing so much more than we realise. But in order for them to function at optimal capacity we have to fuel them adequately. By eating the right types of food before, during and after exercise you can influence your energy levels and help prepare your body for the demands of your workout and subsequent recovery from it. Individual nutritional needs will, of course, vary depending on your ability and the intensity of the activity, but the general rules are the same and you can tailor them to your needs. When exercising, it is even more important to ensure you are eating quality, non-processed food. Real, unprocessed foods will have a larger amount of the nutrients your body needs, compared to processed foods, and these nutrients play a vital role in preparing and repairing your body before and after exercise. These principles are straightforward and simple, but they are core to this book and to Mindful Chef's beliefs.

WHAT SHOULD I EAT BEFORE AND AFTER EXERCISE?

When I worked as a trainer this was always the question I was asked most. Pre-exercise nutrition is really important. Eating before exercise helps to boost energy, preserve muscle mass and aids recovery during and after training.

If I have planned my day properly I'll usually eat a full meal, consisting of proteins, carbohydrates and fats, about 2 hours before I train. The protein will help maintain or increase lean muscle mass; the carbohydrates will help fuel my session and give me the energy I need to train – they will also help stimulate the release of insulin, which is important when training to improve protein synthesis and maintain muscle. Having fats in your meal won't actually fuel your workout (unless you are participating in low-level intensity exercise where the aerobic system is dominant), but they do slow digestion, which can help your glucose levels remain stable.

If I haven't had time to eat a full meal or I don't have much time before training (say less than 60 minutes), I will usually make a shake consisting of protein powder, banana, berries, nut butter and water. If I don't have time to prepare anything and have to grab something quickly, my favourite on-the-go option is usually sliced meat and a handful of berries, or a tin of tuna, some cooked lentils and some fruit.

WHAT ABOUT KEEPING UP MY ENERGY DURING MY WORKOUT?

Nutrition during exercise is very important but only when used in the right circumstances. For elite or endurance athletes it is one of the key factors they need to take into consideration when planning their training. However, if you're a normal person like me and you're just doing a 45-minute HIIT session or attending a class, it's more than likely you won't need an energy drink to fuel your training session. It could actually be doing you more harm than good.

I remember being invited to a summit in Barcelona for a well-known sports drink company who were actively putting together a campaign to highlight and educate consumers on when they should be using their sports drinks and when they shouldn't. Regular exercisers are unlikely to need to replace energy to such a level, so a sports drink isn't recommended during a workout because the carbohydrates used to provide fuel are unnecessary. I would rather stay hydrated with water and ensure that the meals I eat before and after training are full of healthy, non-processed ingredients, to provide my body with all the vitamins, minerals and fibre it needs to help build muscle, recover and supply energy.

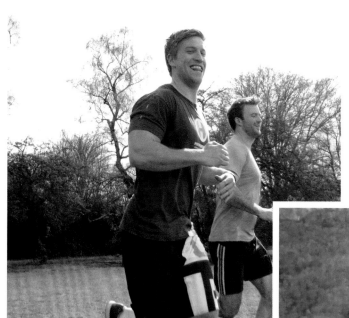

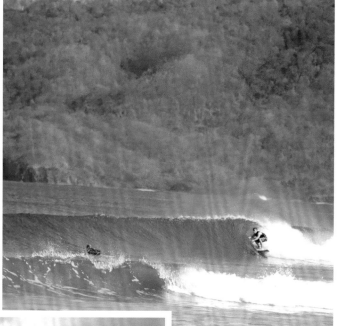

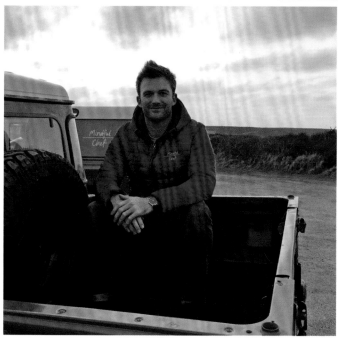

We all have different nutritional requirements, and the amount of food I eat may be very different to the amount Giles eats. However, our guidelines and principles remain the same and can be followed by anyone.

SO WHAT SHOULD I EAT AFTER EXERCISE?

Eating after exercise is very important if you really want to look and feel your best. Eating the right foods will help your body recover, refuel and build lean muscle, as well as provide it with all the vitamins and minerals it needs to perform all of its essential processes after training. Some people think they need to drink a protein shake as soon as they finish a workout, but this isn't always the case. The timing of your shake or meal following training should take into account when you had your previous meal. If it was several hours before you trained, you should be slightly more concerned about eating sooner rather than later. If however, it was closer to training, then as long as you eat within a 2-hour window it will help keep recovery at an optimal level.

Having protein in your post-workout meal is very important, as it will stop any breakdown of muscle and help protein synthesis – both of which will help to maintain or increase lean muscle. As we get older we lose muscle a lot quicker, so it is important to maintain it as much as possible in order to stay strong as we age. Having more lean muscle also makes the body appear firmer. And for anyone worried about bulking up and looking like the Hulk, you shouldn't be. It is very hard to put on a lot of muscle and even harder for women to do so. Sure it can be done, but women have to work much harder than men to achieve this because of different hormonal profiles.

Eating carbohydrates after exercise helps to restore levels of glycogen, which is used for energy during training. Carbohydrates will also help with recovery and preparing you for your next training session. There has been debate in the past about eating fats in post-workout meals, but I believe the benefits outweigh any concerns. Generally people don't like to eat fats after training, as they think it will slow the breakdown and absorption of protein and carbohydrates (which are needed for all of the reasons above). However, there is evidence questioning how important the speed of digestion and absorption of proteins and carbohydrates really is, especially if you have eaten well before training. We think that fats are a great source of energy; they help form cell membranes and aid the delivery of fat-soluble vitamins, therefore they are important for everyone trying to recover from any form of exercise.

We all have different nutritional requirements, and the amount of food I eat may be very different to the amount Giles eats. However, our guidelines and principles remain the same and can be followed by anyone. We encourage everyone to eat real, wholesome, natural food and to try to avoid processed foods as much as possible. I would suggest that you concentrate on the qualith and types of food you are eating to ensure you have a varied diet of protein, carbohydrates and fats. Once you have these basic steps covered, you can start thinking about pre- and post-exercise nutrition. We want everyone to provide their bodies with the best-quality produce and ingredients to help them recover, build lean muscle and increase their energy levels. If you manage to do this you will feel more energised and be a more productive person, and this will benefit all areas of your life, helping you be the best version of you possible.

HERE ARE SOME OF MY FAVOURITE MEALS AFTER TRAINING:

- Mexican veggie chilli with sweet potato nachos & guacamole (see page 152)
- Indian chicken curry with roasted sweet potato & wild rice (see page 160)
- Creamy garlic mushroom & lentil ragù with sweet potato noodles (see page 169)

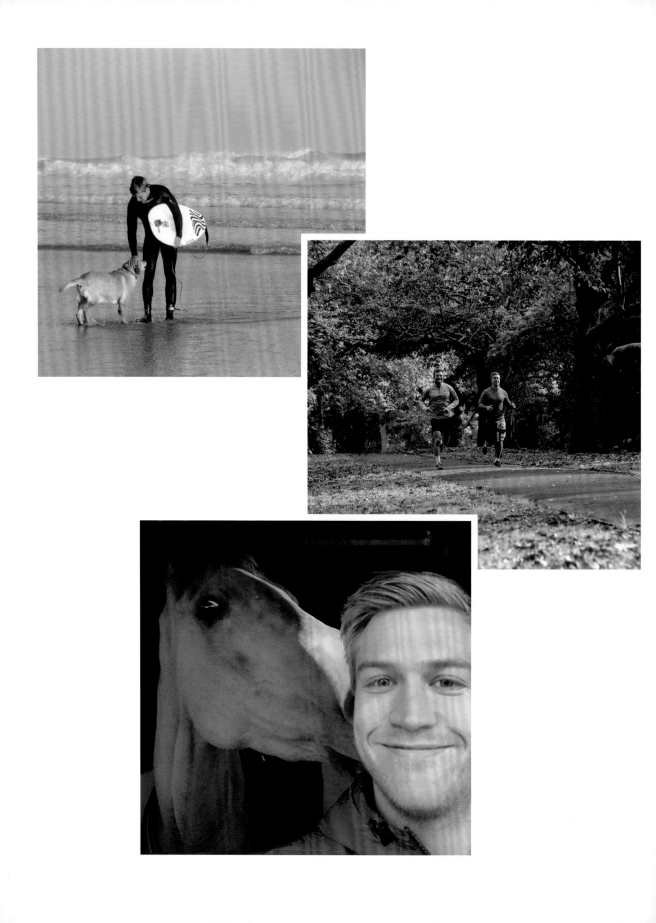

TOP TIPS FOR EXERCISE AND NUTRITION

1. **WHEN TO REFUEL**

   Pre-exercise nutrition should give you enough energy for your session and help retain lean muscle mass. Nutrition during exercise will help you stay hydrated and provide energy to finish the task at hand. Nutrition post-exercise will help your body recover, refuel and build lean muscle mass.

2. **BALANCE YOUR MACRONUTRIENTS**

   A winning combination of quality proteins, carbohydrates and fats will give you all the nutrients, fibre and minerals you need to perform at your best.

3. **PLAN YOUR WEEK!**

   On days when you are training it is vitally important that you have food both before and after your workout. If that means you have to prepare it the night before or at the weekend, try to take some time to do so. Remember, eating before training will help you perform at your best. The more energy you have, the harder you will be able to train and the more you will be able to get out of your body. Eating after training will help you recover from a hard session and prepare you for the next one, so it really will help you achieve your goals if you are prepared, rather than grabbing the easiest option.

4. **REPLACE LOST FLUIDS AFTER EXERCISE**

   Exercise is hard, and we sweat to help regulate body temperature. Following training it is essential to replace this lost water, and our muscles cannot fully recover unless they are properly hydrated. During exercise we need water to deliver oxygen and nutrients around the body. Remember, unless you are an elite athlete or training for longer than 90 minutes, you probably don't need a sports drink.

All the recipes in this chapter have been included because they provide a healthy amount of protein and carbohydrates, which our bodies need pre- and post-training to ensure we are able to train at our best and recover fully before the next session.

Our spicy veggie chilli is packed with filling kidney beans, an excellent source of protein and fibre, and served with sweet potato nachos and homemade guacamole. The sweet potato nachos are a delicious snack in their own right – they taste amazing and are a much healthier alternative to salty fried tortilla chips. You could spoon over some fresh tomato and chilli salsa to add even more flavour!

MEXICAN VEGGIE CHILLI WITH SWEET POTATO NACHOS & GUACAMOLE

1 red onion
140g courgettes
2 garlic cloves
300g sweet potatoes
coconut or olive oil
240g drained kidney beans
300g tinned chopped tomatoes
1 tsp chilli flakes
1 avocado
juice of 1 lime
20g creamed coconut
40ml boiling water
sea salt and black pepper

1 Preheat the oven to 200°C/gas mark 6.

2 Finely dice the onion and courgettes and finely chop the garlic.

3 Peel and thinly slice the sweet potatoes. Toss with ½ tablespoon of oil and season with sea salt. Place the slices of sweet potato in a baking tray and bake in the oven for 15–20 minutes, turning halfway through.

4 Heat 1 teaspoon of oil in a medium-sized pan and fry the garlic and onion for 3 minutes, then add the courgettes and fry for a further 5 minutes.

5 Add the drained beans, chopped tomatoes and chilli flakes and simmer on a gentle heat for 10 minutes, until the sauce has thickened. Season with sea salt and black pepper.

6 Peel and de-stone the avocado and place it in a bowl with half the lime juice. Roughly mash the avocado with the back of a fork.

7 To make the coconut sauce, mix the creamed coconut with the boiling water in a bowl.

8 To serve, spoon the veggie chilli on to warm plates. Place the sweet potato nachos alongside and spoon over the crushed avocado, then drizzle over the coconut sauce and the remaining lime juice.

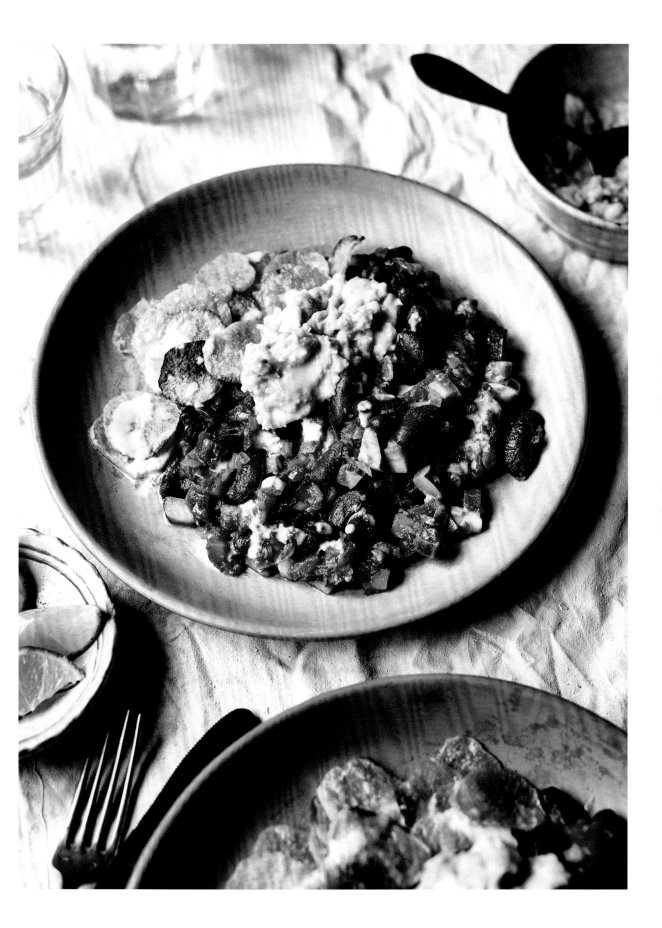

This soft comforting winter warmer is topped with sweet roasted parsnip crisps that give the dish a lovely crunch. It's drizzled with a vibrant, chunky homemade pesto made with olive oil, freshly chopped parsley and walnuts, which contain alpha-linolenic acid to help reduce bad cholesterol.

PARSNIP, KALE & KIDNEY BEAN HOTPOT WITH PARSLEY & WALNUT PESTO

2 garlic cloves
1 aubergine
40g kale
300g parsnips
olive oil
240g drained kidney beans
400g tinned chopped tomatoes
1 vegetable stock cube
handful of fresh flat-leaf parsley
20g walnuts
juice of ½ lemon
sea salt and black pepper

1 Preheat the oven to 200°C/gas mark 6.

2 Finely chop the garlic. Chop the aubergine into 2cm pieces and roughly chop the kale. Peel the parsnips and very thinly slice into rounds.

3 Place the parsnips on a baking tray with 2 teaspoons of oil and a pinch of sea salt. Roast in the oven for 20 minutes, turning halfway, until beginning to crisp.

4 Heat 1 teaspoon of oil in a large pan on a medium heat. Add the aubergine and half the garlic and cook for 7 minutes, until softened.

5 Add the drained kidney beans and the chopped tomatoes and mix in the stock cube. Simmer for 5 minutes, then add the kale for a further 5 minutes.

6 Meanwhile, to make the parsley and walnut pesto, finely chop the parsley and the walnuts and mix with the rest of the garlic, 1 tablespoon of olive oil and the lemon juice. Season with sea salt and black pepper.

7 To serve, spoon the kidney bean hotpot on to warm plates, and top with a layer of parsnip crisps. Drizzle over the parsley and walnut pesto.

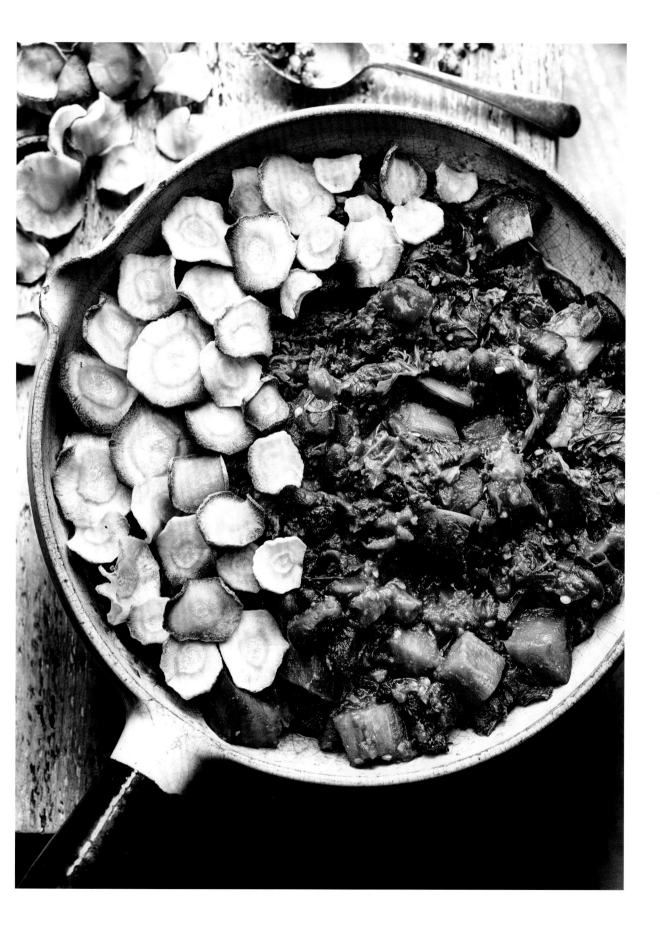

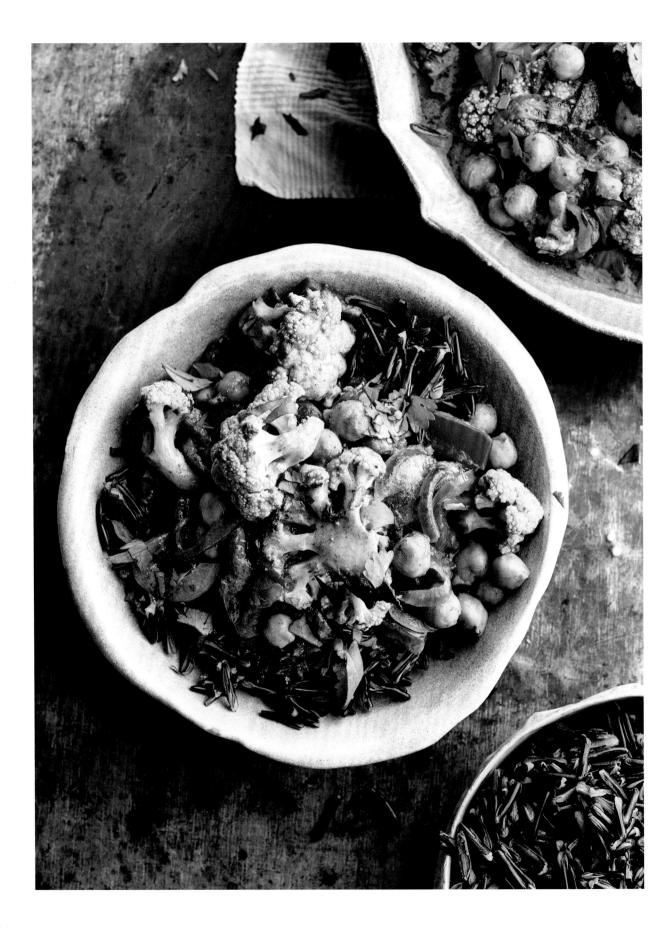

We've used a nutty tikka masala paste to bring bags of flavour to this veggie curry. Roasting cauliflower is a delicious way to bring out its flavour; it gives the florets a crisp exterior yet they remain tender on the inside. Cauliflower is so versatile and with its ability to aid cell detoxification it's a nourishing vegetable that is worth including regularly in your diet.

ROASTED CAULIFLOWER & CHICKPEA TIKKA MASALA WITH WILD RICE

100g wild rice
500ml boiling water
½ cauliflower
coconut or olive oil
1 red onion
2 tomatoes
handful of fresh coriander
2 tbsp tikka masala paste
200g drained chickpeas
200ml coconut milk
sea salt

1 Preheat the oven to 200°C/gas mark 6.

2 Place the wild rice in a pan with the boiling water and a pinch of sea salt and simmer for 25–30 minutes, until the rice is cooked.

3 Cut the cauliflower into small florets, place in a bowl and mix with 1 teaspoon of oil and a sprinkle of sea salt. Place on a baking tray and roast in the oven for 10–15 minutes, until golden.

4 Meanwhile, thinly slice the red onion. Roughly chop the tomatoes and coriander.

5 Heat ½ teaspoon of oil in a medium-sized pan and cook the red onion for 5 minutes, until softened. Stir in the tikka masala paste and cook for 1 minute, then add the roasted cauliflower florets to the pan and stir to coat in the paste.

6 Add the drained chickpeas to the pan along with the chopped tomatoes, coconut milk and 100ml of water. Bring to the boil, then reduce the heat and simmer for 10 minutes, until the sauce has reduced.

7 Stir in half the coriander leaves. Drain the wild rice.

8 To serve, place the rice on warm plates and spoon over the cauliflower and chickpea masala. Sprinkle over the remaining coriander.

The wealth of omega-3 fatty acids found in salmon can aid muscle recovery, so this is a great dish to enjoy after a big workout. The brown rice adds plenty of of fibre, and its bran, which is the outer layer of the grain, can help lower cholesterol, keeping the heart healthy. The crunchy slaw is a vitamin-packed rainbow of veg.

HONEY & GINGER SALMON SKEWERS WITH RAINBOW SLAW & BROWN RICE

80g brown rice
400ml boiling water
4cm fresh ginger
1 tbsp honey
2 tbsp tamari
juice of 1 lime
300g salmon fillets
150g carrots
50g radishes
80g sugar snap peas
coconut or olive oil
sea salt

1 Rinse the brown rice and place it in a pan with the boiling water. Add a pinch of sea salt and simmer for 20–25 minutes, until the rice is tender.

2 Peel and finely chop the ginger. In a bowl, mix together the honey, tamari, ginger and half the lime juice. Place half this mixture in a separate bowl. Cut the salmon fillets into bite-sized pieces (around 2cm) and place in one of the bowls of sauce to marinate for 10 minutes while you prepare the salad.

3 To make the slaw, peel the carrots and cut into matchsticks (or use a julienne peeler or spiraliser if you have one). Slice the radishes and sugar snaps into matchsticks. Place in a bowl and drizzle over ½ tablespoon of oil and the rest of the lime juice.

4 Thread the salmon pieces on to the skewers.

5 Heat a griddle pan on a medium-high heat and add 1 tablespoon of oil (make sure the pan is well oiled to prevent sticking). Add the salmon skewers and cook for 10–15 minutes, turning every 2–3 minutes, until the salmon is cooked through.

6 Drain the brown rice.

7 Spoon the rice on to warm plates, top each one with 2 salmon skewers and serve the rainbow slaw alongside. Drizzle the remaining sauce over the salad and skewers.

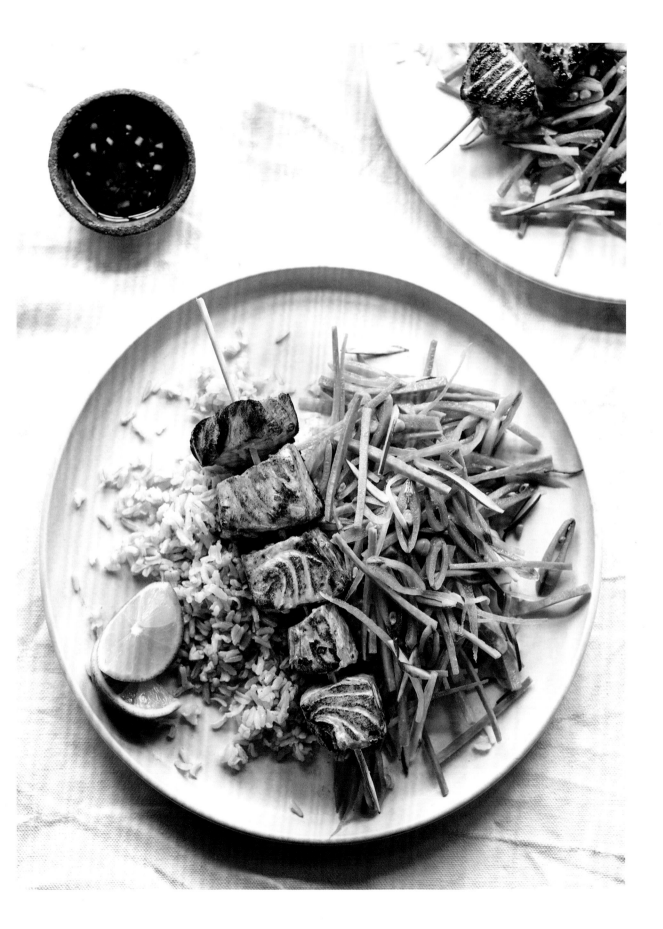

This creamy, earthy Indian curry is guaranteed to warm you up on a chilly winter's day. It's spiced with aromatic garam masala, a staple combination of spices in Indian cooking, which traditionally includes ground coriander, cumin, cinnamon, black pepper, nutmeg, cardamom and cloves – a great mix for fighting off winter colds. The sweet potato adds a beta-carotene boost for strengthening the immune system.

INDIAN CHICKEN CURRY WITH ROASTED SWEET POTATO & WILD RICE

80g wild rice
400ml boiling water
4cm fresh ginger
2 garlic cloves
1 red onion
160g sweet potatoes
2 x 170g chicken breasts
coconut oil
2 tsp garam masala
1 tsp turmeric
200ml coconut milk
80g spinach
sea salt and black pepper

1 Preheat the oven to 180°C/gas mark 4.

2 Rinse the wild rice and put it into a saucepan with the boiling water and a pinch of sea salt. Simmer for 25–30 minutes, then drain.

3 Peel and finely chop the ginger. Finely chop the garlic and finely slice the red onion. Peel the sweet potatoes and cut into 1cm cubes. Thinly slice the chicken breasts.

4 Place the sweet potatoes on a baking tray and toss with 1 tablespoon of oil and a sprinkle of sea salt. Roast in the oven for 15 minutes, turning halfway through cooking.

5 Meanwhile, heat 1 tablespoon of oil in a large pan on a medium heat and fry the onion, garlic and ginger for 3 minutes. Add the garam masala and the chicken and fry for 8 minutes, until golden brown.

6 Stir in the turmeric and the coconut milk, season with sea salt and black pepper and simmer for 10 minutes, until the chicken is cooked through. Stir in the spinach and the roasted sweet potato for the last 2 minutes.

7 Serve the curry in warm bowls with the wild rice.

Wild garlic is in season from April to May in the UK, when there is an abundance of it. We love chopping it finely chopped and mixing it with a glug of olive oil and chopped pine nuts to make our own homemade pesto. You can buy wild garlic from specialist stores or forage for it yourself in woodland areas – you'll know when you're near it –the aroma is hard to miss!

WILD GARLIC PESTO BAKED CHICKEN WITH CARROT MASH & TENDERSTEM

20g wild garlic leaves
30g pine nuts
olive oil
juice of ½ a lemon
2 x 170g chicken breasts
400g carrots
200g tenderstem broccoli
180g cherry tomatoes
sea salt and black pepper

1 Preheat the oven to 200°C/gas mark 6.

2 To make the wild garlic pesto, finely chop the wild garlic leaves and roughly chop the pine nuts. Place in a bowl and mix in 1 tablespoon of olive oil and the lemon juice. Season with salt and pepper.

3 Put the chicken breasts into an ovenproof dish and cover with a layer of the pesto. Bake in the oven for 25 minutes, or until cooked through.

4 Meanwhile, peel the carrots and chop them into 1cm pieces. Place in a saucepan of boiling water and simmer for 20 minutes, until soft.

5 Trim the tenderstem broccoli. Place the tenderstem, tomatoes and the remaining pine nuts on a baking tray, drizzle over 1½ tablespoons of oil, and roast in the oven for 10 minutes.

6 Drain the carrots and mash with a potato masher. Season with salt and pepper.

7 To serve, spoon the carrot mash on to plates. Cut the chicken into slices. Place the sliced chicken on top of the carrot mash and serve with the tenderstem, tomatoes and pine nuts.

Inspired by the Singaporean classic, these bright spiced sweet potato noodles are so delicious we could eat this every week. We poach the chicken breasts to keep them moist, before shredding them with a fork. Sugar snaps have edible pods, unlike most other pea pods, and are delicious stir-fried so that they still have their sweet, crisp bite.

SINGAPORE-STYLE SWEET POTATO NOODLES WITH SHREDDED CHICKEN

4cm fresh ginger
2 garlic cloves
1 red pepper
400g sweet potatoes
1 chicken stock cube
500ml boiling water
2 x 170g chicken breasts
1 tbsp medium curry powder
80g sugar snap peas
2 tbsp tamari
juice of 1 lime

1 Peel and finely chop the ginger and crush or finely chop the garlic. Thinly slice the red pepper.

2 Peel the sweet potatoes. Prepare the sweet potato noodles using a peeler and slice into long thin strips (or use a julienne peeler or a spiraliser, if you have one).

3 Dissolve the stock cube in the boiling water, then pour into a small saucepan and bring back to the boil. Add the chicken breasts, ensuring they are covered in stock (add more boiling water if needed). Cover the pan, reduce the heat and simmer for 15 minutes, or until the chicken is cooked through.

4 Meanwhile, heat ½ tablespoon of oil in a wok (or frying pan) on a medium heat. Add the noodles and cook for 8–10 minutes, until softened. Remove and keep warm.

5 Using two forks, shred the poached chicken into small pieces.

6 Heat another ½ tablespoon of oil in the same wok (or frying pan).

7 Add the garlic, ginger and curry powder and stir for 1 minute, then add the red pepper and sugar snaps and cook for 4 minutes. Add the tamari, chicken, half the lime juice and the noodles and stir and cook for 2 minutes.

8 Serve in warm bowls and drizzle over the remaining lime juice.

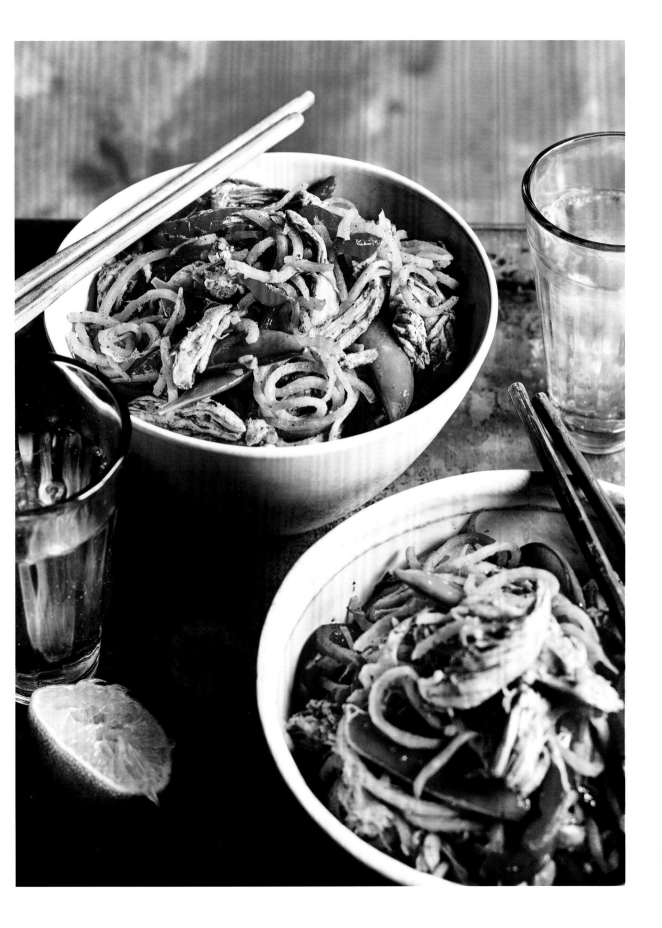

Drawing inspiration from the traditional Indonesian nasi goreng, a popular breakfast dish, we've swapped white rice for brown and have topped it with a fried egg for a healthy dose of omega-3 fatty acids.

NASI GORENG WITH PORK, EGG, CARROT RIBBONS & BROWN RICE

80g brown rice
400ml boiling water
40g spinach
1 red chilli
4cm fresh ginger
2 tbsp tamari
1 tbsp sesame oil
300g pork fillet
200g carrots
juice of 1 lime
coconut oil
2 eggs
sea salt

1 Rinse the brown rice and put it into a saucepan with the boiling water and a pinch of sea salt. Simmer for 20–25 minutes. In the last 2 minutes of cooking the rice, add the spinach to the pan, then drain.

2 Meanwhile, to make the marinade, finely chop the red chilli and peel and finely chop the ginger. Place the chilli and ginger in a bowl with the tamari and sesame oil and mix well.

3 Slice the pork fillet very thinly and add to the marinade. Stir to coat, then leave for 5 minutes to marinate.

4 Peel the carrots. Using a peeler, slice them into long thin ribbons.

5 Heat a frying pan on a medium heat. Add the pork and the marinade to the pan and cook for 6 minutes, stirring occasionally. Then add the carrot ribbons and half the lime juice and fry for 2–3 minutes, until the pork is cooked through. Remove the pork and the carrot ribbons from the pan and keep warm.

6 Heat 1 teaspoon of oil in the same frying pan and fry the eggs for a few minutes, until cooked.

7 To serve, spoon the pork and carrot ribbons on to warm plates alongside the spinach rice. Drizzle over the remaining lime juice and top each plate with a fried egg.

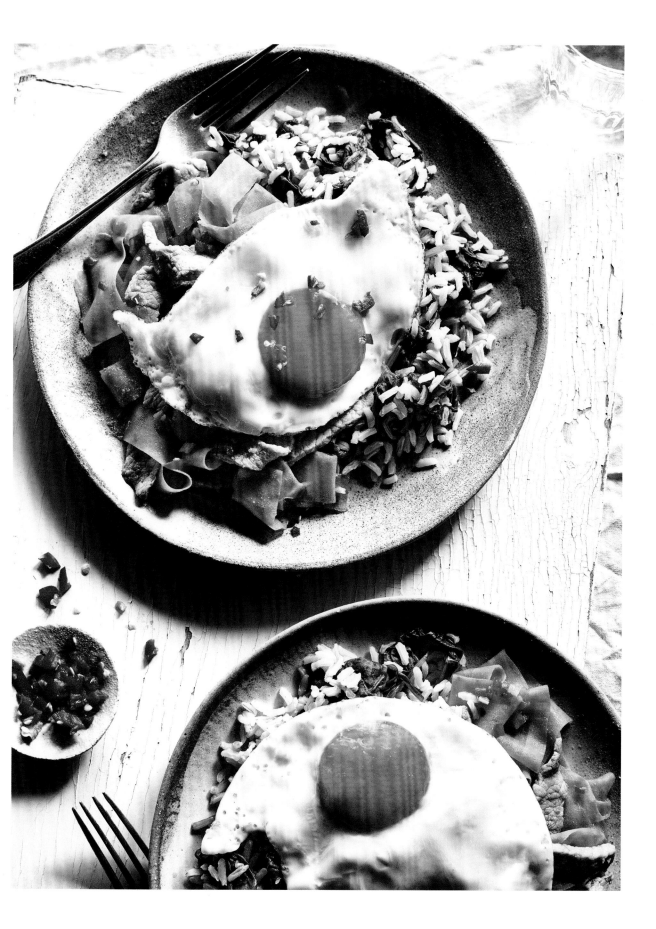

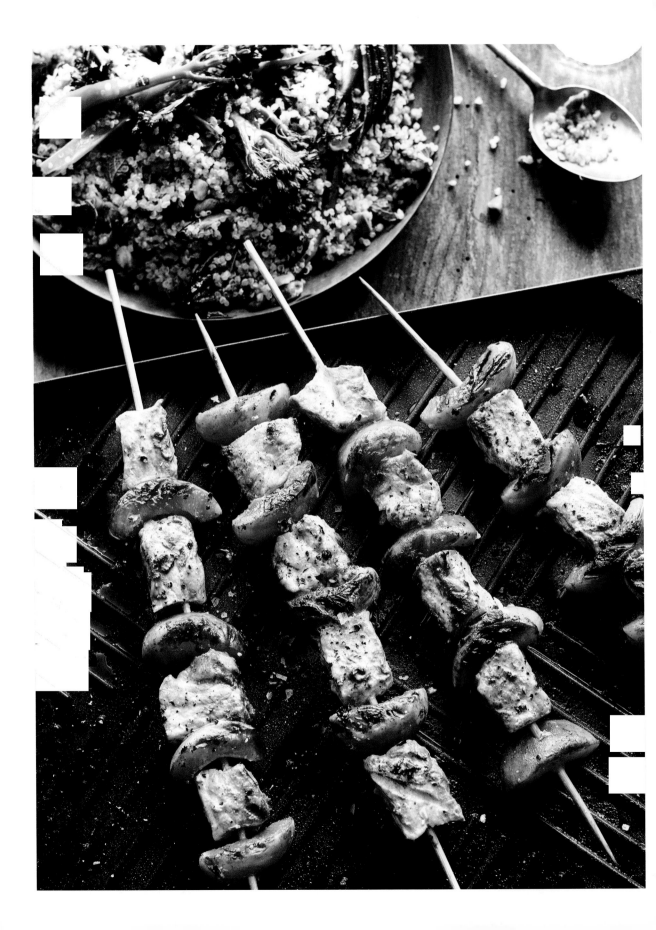

This is a fantastic dish for a barbecue – sweet ripe apricots are paired with juicy pork to make delicious caramelised kebabs. Perfect for grilling over charcoal, the kebabs can also be cooked quickly and easily on a griddle pan if the British summer isn't kind to us. We've added crunchy pistachios to the quinoa, which give it a rich nuttiness, while adding a wealth of minerals, and have tossed through some chopped mint leaves for soothing the stomach. The vitamin C from the apricots helps maintain a healthy immune system.

PORK & APRICOT KEBABS WITH PISTACHIO & MINT QUINOA

4 fresh apricots
120g tenderstem broccoli
1 red onion
handful of fresh mint
coconut or olive oil
80g quinoa
300ml boiling water
2 x 150g pork loin steaks
15g pistachios
juice of 1 lemon
sea salt and black pepper

1 Preheat the oven to 200°C/gas mark 6.

2 Slice the apricots into quarters and take out the stones. Trim the tenderstem and slice the red onion into chunks. Roughly chop the mint leaves.

3 Place the red onion on a baking tray, drizzle over 1 teaspoon of oil and place in the oven for 20 minutes. Halfway through the cooking time, add the tenderstem to the baking tray along with another tablespoon of oil and return to the oven for 10 minutes.

4 Rinse the quinoa and place in a saucepan with the boiling water. Add a pinch of sea salt, then simmer for 15 minutes, until cooked.

5 Slice each pork loin steak into 8 bite-sized pieces. Take 4 skewers and thread 4 pieces of pork and 4 apricot quarters on to each one. Drizzle over ½ tablespoon of oil and sprinkle with salt and pepper.

6 Preheat a griddle pan (or barbecue). Add the pork and apricot skewers and cook for 15 minutes, turning every 3–4 minutes, until the pork is cooked through.

7 Drain the quinoa, then stir in the roasted onions, tenderstem, mint leaves, pistachios and half the lemon juice.

8 Spoon the quinoa on to plates and serve the kebabs alongside, drizzled with the rest of the lemon juice.

When buying red meat, we recommend buying grass-fed (for more on this, see page 17). Beef is loaded with iron, zinc and B vitamins for combating fatigue, and the delicious blend of Thai ingredients adds even more health-giving properties to this dish. Red chilli boosts digestion, while the zingy ginger helps to reduce inflammation, making this a great post-workout meal.

THAI-STYLE SPICY BEEF WITH TENDERSTEM & BROWN RICE

80g brown rice
400ml boiling water
1 fresh lemongrass stalk
1 fresh red chilli
4cm fresh ginger
200g tenderstem broccoli
1 yellow pepper
30g cashew nuts
2 x 170g beef steaks
juice of 1 lime
2 tbsp tamari
2 tbsp fish sauce
2 tsp honey
coconut oil
sea salt

1 Rinse the brown rice, then put it into a saucepan with the boiling water and a pinch of salt and simmer for 20–25 minutes.

2 Meanwhile, trim the ends of the lemongrass, remove the outer layer and finely chop. Finely slice the red chilli (remove the seeds for less heat if preferred). Peel and finely grate or chop the ginger. Trim the tenderstem and slice in half lengthways. Thinly slice the yellow pepper. Roughly chop or crush the cashew nuts. Thinly slice the beef steaks.

3 To make the spicy Thai sauce, mix the lime juice, tamari, fish sauce, honey and sliced chilli together in a bowl.

4 Heat 1 tablespoon of oil in a large pan on a medium heat and add the lemongrass and ginger. Fry for 2 minutes, then add the steak strips and fry for 3 minutes. Add the tenderstem and yellow pepper and cook for a further 5 minutes.

5 Add the spicy Thai sauce to the pan and cook for 3 minutes. Drain the brown rice.

6 Serve the rice on warm plates, and spoon over the spicy beef, tenderstem and yellow pepper. Sprinkle over the cashew nuts.

This wonderful coconut and garlic mushroom ragù is packed with bone-building kale and antioxidant-rich lentils. It's served on a bed of sweet potato noodles, which are a great partner for the earthy flavours of the chestnut mushrooms. The tahini gives the sauce a lovely richness, and is a great source of vitamin E, which can help strengthen the nervous system.

CREAMY GARLIC MUSHROOM & LENTIL RAGÙ WITH SWEET POTATO NOODLES

2 garlic cloves
1 red onion
120g chestnut mushrooms
60g kale
handful of fresh basil
40g creamed coconut
150ml boiling water
350g sweet potatoes
coconut oil or olive oil
150g cooked lentils (from a tin or pouch)
2 tsp tahini
sea salt and black pepper

1 Finely chop the garlic and thinly slice the red onion and mushrooms. Roughly chop the kale and the basil.

2 Dissolve the creamed coconut in the boiling water.

3 To make the sweet potato noodles, peel the sweet potatoes and then, using a peeler, slice into long thin strips (or use a julienne peeler or spiraliser).

4 Heat ½ tablespoon of oil in a medium-sized pan on a medium heat and fry the garlic and red onion for 5 minutes. Season with sea salt and black pepper. Add the mushrooms and cook for 3 minutes, until softened.

6 Drain and rinse the lentils, then add to the mushrooms and cook for 2 minutes. Lower the heat, add the creamed coconut and the kale and cook for 10 minutes, until the sauce has reduced. Stir in the tahini and half the basil leaves.

7 Meanwhile, heat ½ tablespoon of oil in a frying pan on a medium heat and cook the sweet potato noodles for 8–10 minutes, until softened and turning golden.

8 Serve the sweet potato noodles on warm plates, and spoon over the creamy garlic mushroom and lentil ragù. Sprinkle over the remaining basil leaves.

This juicy burger is made with sun-dried tomato paste and garlic for a rich flavour, and is paired with steamed spinach and an oozing poached egg. As well as being a great side to this burger, the crunchy beetroot and parsnip crisps make a nutritious snack. Beetroot is a wonderfully nourishing vegetable, and with its high levels of iron and antioxidants it helps detox the liver and purify the blood. This super root veg can also stimulate red blood cells, therefore increasing oxygen uptake, and in large quantities has been known to improve athletic endurance.

BEEF BURGER WITH POACHED EGG, SPINACH & BEETROOT CRISPS

1 garlic clove
200g beetroots
200g parsnips
few sprigs of fresh thyme
coconut or olive oil
300g beef mince
2 tbsp sun-dried tomato paste
120g baby vine tomatoes
80g spinach
2 eggs
sea salt and black pepper

1 Preheat the oven to 200°C/gas mark 6.

2 Finely chop the garlic. Peel and finely slice the beetroots and the parsnips. Spread the sliced vegetables out on a baking tray, sprinkle over the thyme leaves and a pinch of salt and drizzle over ½ tablespoon of oil. Place in the oven for 10–15 minutes, turning halfway through.

3 In a bowl, mix the beef mince with the garlic and sun-dried tomato paste. Form into 2 burgers and season with salt and pepper. Place on one side of a baking tray, and on the other side place the tomatoes with 1 teaspoon of oil. Transfer to the oven for 15 minutes, until cooked.

5 Meanwhile, place the spinach in a steamer over a saucepan of boiling water for 3–4 minutes, until wilted, then set aside and keep warm.

6 Heat another saucepan of water and bring to a gentle simmer. Create a gentle whirlpool in the pan with a spoon, then carefully break the eggs into the middle, one at a time. Cook for 3–4 minutes, until the whites are cooked, then remove from the pan.

7 Place each beef burger on a warm plate, top with spinach and a poached egg, and sprinkle over a pinch of salt. Serve alongside the parsnip and beetroot crisps, and the roasted tomatoes.

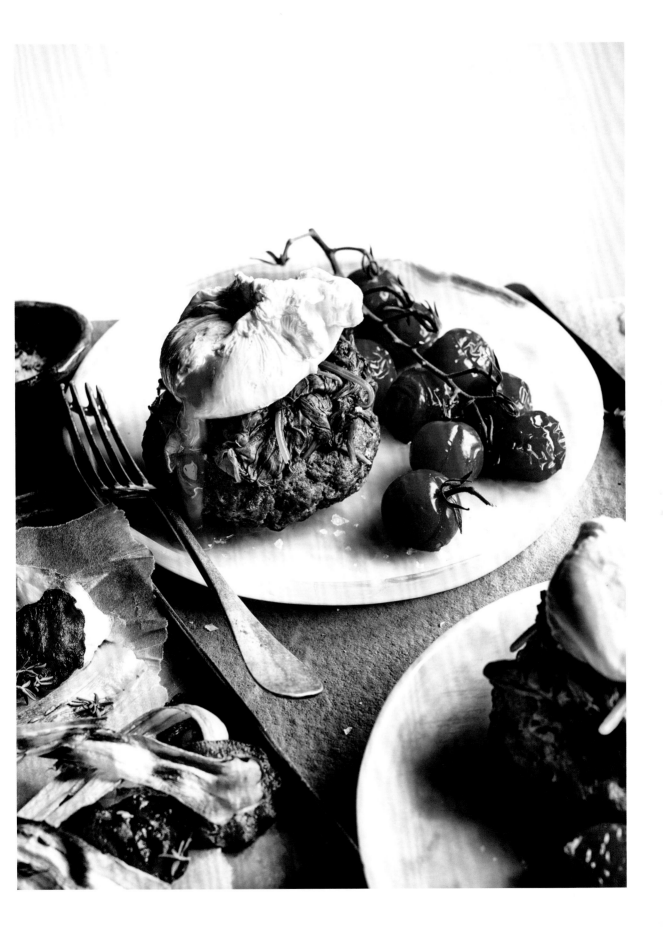

SLEEP

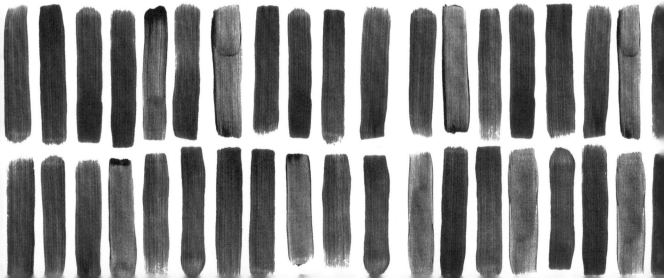

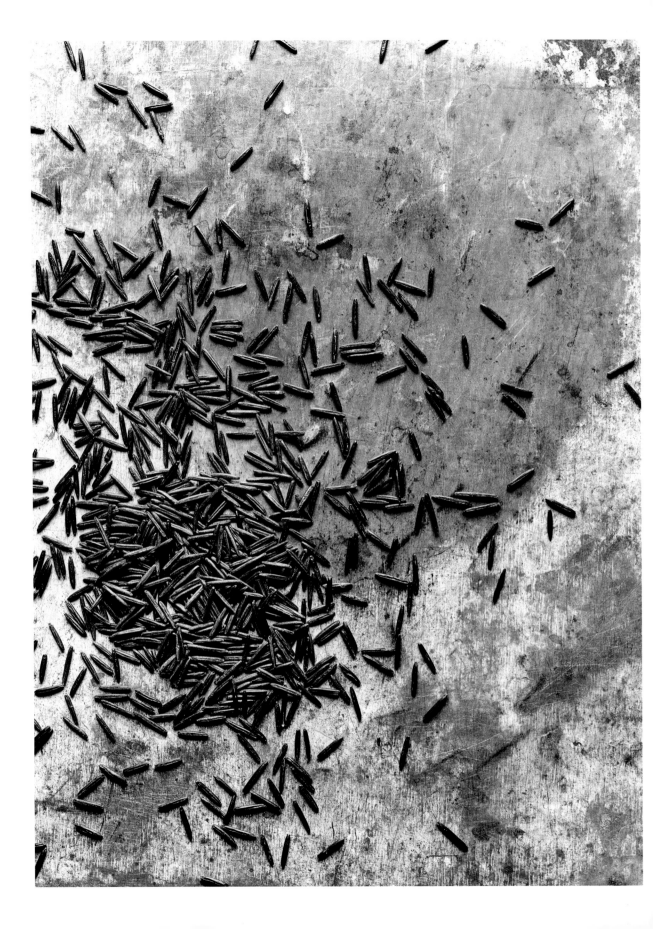

SLEEP

Many people believe food is the most important factor in determining optimal health and well-being. While that may be true, another factor that we often disregard is sleep.

Sleep plays a vital role in both our physical and mental health. During sleep our bodies work to restore muscle and replenish nutrients, support healthy brain function and repair our blood cells to promote physical health. Our immune system relies on sleep to stay healthy, and if we don't get enough sleep we may struggle to fight common infections. In some cases sleep deficiency can even increase the risk of chronic health problems.

While we should definitely be concerned with the types of food we eat during the day to give us enough energy to perform, the right foods can also help us sleep better. And if we enter a regular sleeping pattern, where we experience a deeper state of sleep, and have at least eight hours of sleep a night, we are in turn able to improve our health.

So why is food so important for sleep? Well, in order to obtain good sleep you should have a varied diet that has a healthy balance of proteins, carbohydrates and fats. The more varied your diet, the more micronutrients like minerals, vitamins and antioxidants you will be able to provide for your body. This will help your body to perform all the functions it needs to while sleep is taking place and will ultimately help you to wake up feeling fresher and more energised. With this in mind, all our recipes have been carefully designed to provide a variety of nutrients essential to help your body perform optimally.

The more varied your diet, the more micronutrients like minerals, vitamins and antioxidants you will be able to provide for your body

However, there are also some specific foods you can eat in the evening that will help you get a better night's sleep; they have in fact been proven to be sleep promoters. A good example of this is foods that contain an amino acid called tryptophan. Tryptophan is found in foods such as chicken, nuts and seeds; it helps boost the sleep-inducing hormone melatonin.

- **B VITAMINS**

    These help regulate tryptophan levels, so ensuring that you aren't deficient in any of them can help promote good sleep. Good examples of foods that contain higher levels of B vitamins are broccoli, lentils and tuna. Vitamin B9 (folic acid) deficiency has also been linked to insomnia. Avocados are a great source of vitamin B9.

- **CALCIUM**

    When found in abundance in the body, calcium helps us to relax, so it follows that if we have enough in our bodies it can help us with sleep. Foods rich in calcium are leafy green vegetables, broccoli and beans. Many of you reading this will wonder why we don't suggest using dairy to increase calcium levels, as it seems the most obvious choice. All of our meals are dairy free, and we choose to omit dairy products because we believe there are better food sources for calcium. In recent years the dairy industry in the UK has grown exponentially and as a result of this there has been a decline, for the most part, in the quality of milk and other dairy products. Due to the demand for milk, its production methods have diminished in quality, resulting in an inferior product and one we don't want to give our customers. We also try to cater for as many people as possible, and as there are now lots of people suffering from lactose intolerance (a result of the gut not being able to digest lactose properly), we prefer to ensure everyone has an opportunity to eat great-tasting, healthy food.

- **MAGNESIUM**

    Magnesium plays a vital role in energy production and muscle relaxation and can help reduce our levels of cortisol (for more on this, see page 58). While taking more magnesium won't guarantee a great night's sleep, being deficient in it will guarantee you don't sleep well. Luckily for us, magnesium is found in lots of food sources so it's difficult to have low levels. Foods such as whole grains, avocados, green leafy vegetables, bananas and salmon are just a few of these.

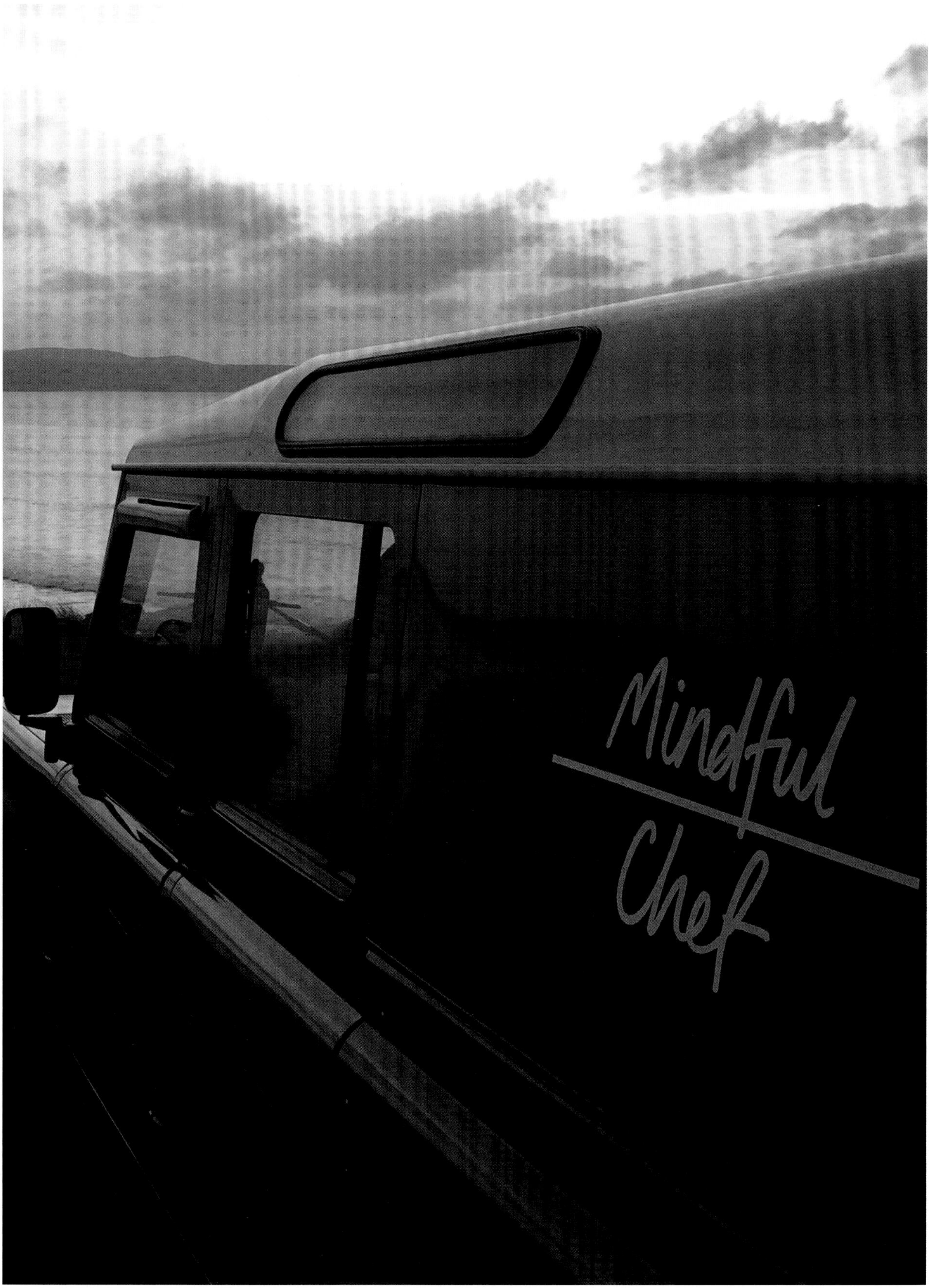
Mindful
Chef

- **VITAMIN D** Finally, vitamin D is also important for getting a good night's sleep. This hormone (that's right, it's actually a hormone rather than a vitamin, as the body produces it itself) helps increase calcium uptake and absorption. We have already seen how calcium helps sleep, so it's important to maintain good levels. The best way to increase your vitamin D levels is to get outside in the sun, but you can also include foods rich in vitamin D in your diet. Foods like eggs and fatty fish such as salmon, tuna and sardines are all good sources of vitamin D.

Some of my favourite meals, like the Spicy Mexican quinoa bowl (see page 184) or our Beef & mustard burger with balsamic onions & rosemary carrot fries (see page 202), are good examples of meals that are high in the above vitamins and minerals.

And finally, on the flip side, certain foods can disturb sleep: simple sugars, additives and preservatives are all culprits. Foods containing these types of sugar can cause a spike in blood sugar levels, which in turn increases energy levels in the body and can lead to restlessness. It's always best to avoid these types of foods but it is particularly important to avoid sugary foods when trying to wind down and prepare for bed, so that your body is not having to contend with a constant spiking and drop in blood sugar levels. We never add any artificial ingredients or flavourings to our recipes and instead choose natural, non-processed whole foods.

FOR A GOOD NIGHT'S SLEEP

BOOST	AVOID
Tryptophan	MSG
B vitamins	Stimulants such as coffee and energy drinks
Calcium	
Magnesium	Spicy food
Vitamin D	Sugary foods

TOP FIVE WAYS TO ENSURE GOOD SLEEP

Food takes energy and time to digest. I prefer eating a couple of hours before going to bed. This has nothing to do with the myths about weight gain but much more to do with digestion and the body's core temperature; digestion elevates this, and it has been proven that we sleep a lot better when our core temperature is lowered. I even have a cold shower before bed to lower my body's temperature and find I get to sleep a lot quicker.

1. **AVOID FOODS WITH ADDITIVES SUCH AS MSG**

    MSG is a potent stimulant found in a lot of takeaway meals. If you fancy a curry or Thai, you can easily make your own healthy versions of these at home. I particularly enjoy our Red Thai chicken curry or Pad thai with courgette noodles (see pages 66 and 93).

2. **AVOID STIMULANTS LIKE COFFEE AND ENERGY DRINKS**

    These affect our hormones and neurotransmitters (signals to the brain) and so they keep us awake. I only have caffeine in the morning and find I sleep a lot better avoiding any form of stimulants in the afternoon.

3. **AVOID SPICY FOODS JUST BEFORE BED**

    While some spicy foods have a host of health benefits, for many they can cause problems for the gastrointestinal tract. Foods that cause discomfort to your gut can be a cause of insomnia as your body struggles to process the foods. By eating foods I know my body is able to process and digest well, I find I am able to get to sleep much quicker and don't have to worry about being kept awake due to acid reflux.

4. **THINK ABOUT YOUR LAST MEAL OF THE DAY**

    Your evening meal should be full of nutrient-dense, high fibre, low-calorie vegetables, protein and healthy fats. Protein helps maintain lean muscle (important for body composition) and appetite control so you don't wake up feeling hungry in the middle of the night. The nutritious vegetables and healthy fats facilitate your body's overnight maintenance and keep it balanced.

All of the meals in this chapter are not only delicious but filling, and provide a perfect amount of protein, carbohydrates and fats to ensure your body is able to perform all the natural functions it needs to while you sleep. While eating an avocado or banana won't necessarily send you into a deep slumber, we believe that by eating a varied diet with foods that contain the vitamins and minerals listed in this chapter you may help to improve your sleep.

ONE CAN'T THINK WELL, LOVE WELL, SLEEP WELL, IF ONE HAS NOT DINED WELL

Virginia Woolf

This delicious vegetarian sushi is made using the ancient grain quinoa instead of rice. The quinoa has a sweet umami flavour from the white miso paste and is wrapped in mineral-rich nori, which is shredded and dried seaweed. The cucumber and radish salad makes a refreshing side and injects even more colour and vitamins into the dish!

SUPERFOOD QUINOA & AVOCADO SUSHI WITH MISO & CUCUMBER SALAD

120g quinoa
400ml boiling water
100g carrots
1 avocado
1 cucumber
2 tbsp sweet white miso paste
2 tsp black sesame seeds
80g radishes
juice of ½ lime
2 nori sheets
2 tbsp tamari
sea salt and black pepper

1 Rinse the quinoa and place in a saucepan with the boiling water and a pinch of salt. Simmer for 15 minutes.

2 Meanwhile, grate the carrots. Peel and de-stone the avocado and slice thinly. Cut half the cucumber into thin batons.

3 Drain the quinoa and stir through half the sweet miso paste and half the black sesame seeds. Leave to cool for 5 minutes.

4 Meanwhile, prepare the salad. Thinly slice the radishes. Using a peeler, slice the rest of the cucumber into thin strips (or use a spiraliser). Put the radishes and cucumber strips into a bowl with the remaining miso and sesame seeds and the lime juice. Set aside.

5 Place a nori sheet on a clean chopping board (or on a sushi mat, if you have one). Spread half the quinoa in a thin layer to the edges of the nori, leaving a 2cm gap at the top.

6 Place half the avocado, the cucumber batons and the grated carrot across the middle of the quinoa widthways. Roll the sushi from the bottom up, ensuring the vegetables are tightly packed in, then wet the top of the nori with a little water to seal. Slice the sushi roll into 8 pieces. Repeat with the remaining nori sheet, quinoa and vegetables.

7 Place the sushi rolls on a plate alongside the cucumber salad. Serve the tamari in a bowl or small dish for dipping.

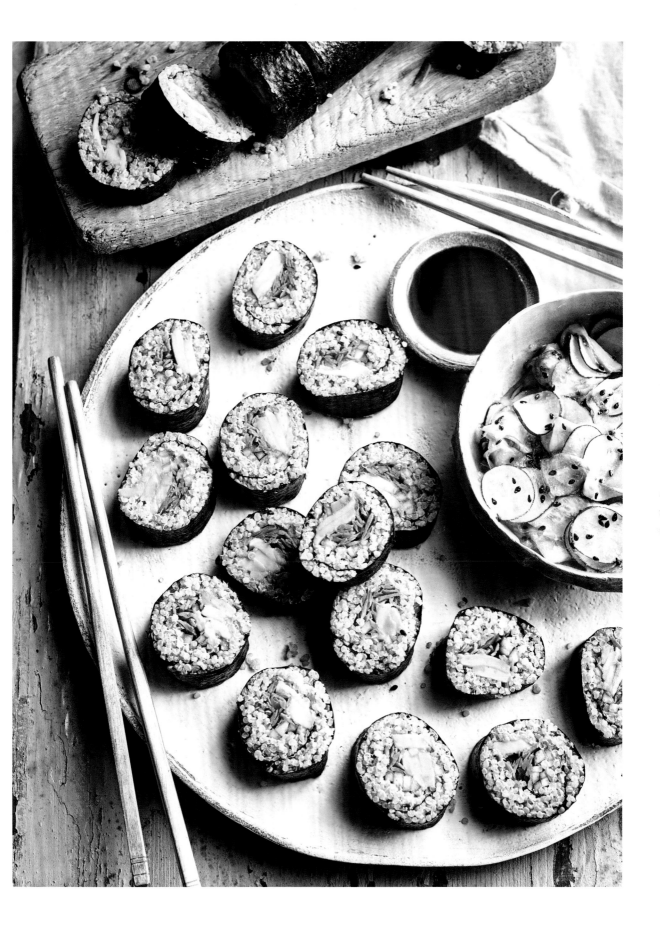

This superfood bowl combines the ancient grain quinoa with punchy jalapeños for a touch of heat, plus fibre-rich kidney beans. Sautéd onion and red pepper is spooned on top, followed by slivers of health-boosting avocado and a swirl of deliciously creamy coconut lime drizzle.

SPICY MEXICAN QUINOA BOWL WITH BEANS & SLICED AVOCADO

80g quinoa
320ml boiling water
1 red onion
1 red pepper
1 avocado
30g pickled sliced jalapeños
a handful of coriander
coconut or olive oil
240g drained kidney beans
2 tsp smoked paprika
20g creamed coconut
juice of 1 lime
sea salt and black pepper

1 Rinse the quinoa and place it in a pan with 300ml of the boiling water. Simmer for 15 minutes until cooked.

2 Meanwhile finely slice the red onion and red pepper. Peel and de-stone the avocado and slice thinly. Roughly chop the jalapeños and the coriander leaves.

3 Heat ½ tablespoon of oil in a medium-sized pan. Add the drained kidney beans to the pan with half the smoked paprika and the jalapeños and cook for 5 minutes. Remove from the pan, set aside and cover.

4 In the same pan, heat ½ tablespoon of oil and fry the onion for 3 minutes, then add the red pepper and fry for 5 minutes. Stir in the rest of the smoked paprika.

5 Meanwhile, in a bowl, mix the creamed coconut with the remaining 20ml of boiling water to make a sauce. Add a squeeze of lime juice and a pinch of sea salt.

6 Drain the quinoa and mix with the kidney beans and half the coriander. Season with sea salt and black pepper.

7 To serve, spoon the quinoa and beans into bowls, top with the red pepper and onion, then layer over the sliced avocado. Drizzle over the coconut lime sauce and scatter over the remaining coriander leaves.

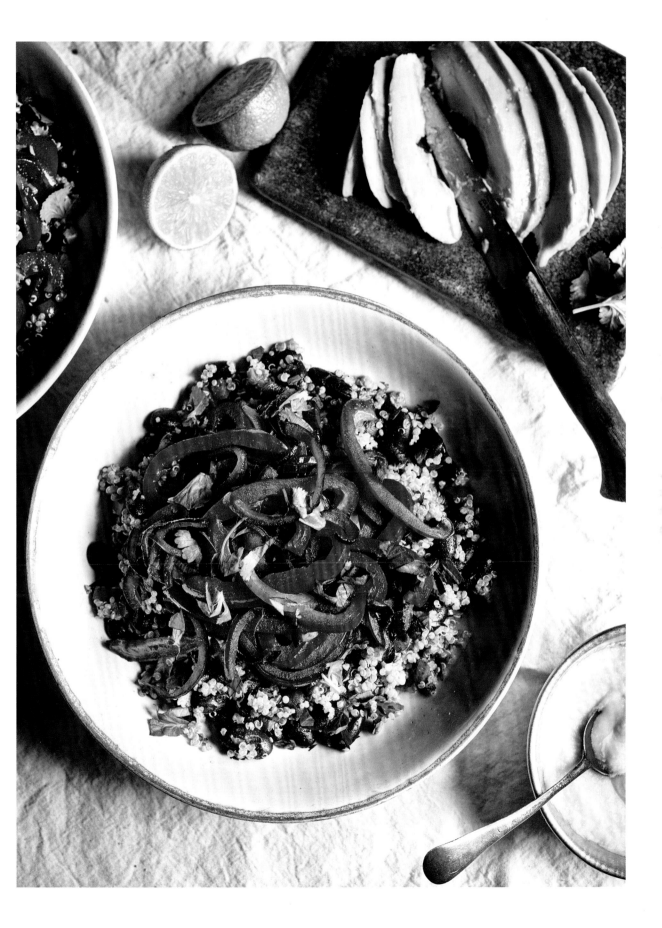

These moreish mini bean burgers have an aubergine 'bun' – which gives your meal an extra dose of vitamins and reduces those heavy carbs. The burgers have a soft texture, and the balsamic vinegar lends them a sweet acidity that will leave you wanting more. The sunflower seeds in the beetroot and rocket salad add a satisfying crunch to the dish and contain vitamin E, for promoting healthy hair and skin.

BEAN BURGERS WITH AUBERGINE, CRUSHED AVOCADO & BEETROOT

2 garlic cloves
1 red onion
1 aubergine
150g beetroot
coconut oil or olive oil
240g drained mixed beans
2 tbsp balsamic vinegar
1 avocado
40g rocket
2 tsp sunflower seeds

1 Preheat the oven to 180°C/gas mark 4.

2 Finely chop the garlic and finely dice the red onion. Slice the aubergine into 5mm thick rounds.

3 Peel the beetroot and chop into 1cm pieces. Place on a baking tray and drizzle with 1 teaspoon of oil. Add a sprinkling of sea salt and place in the oven for 15–20 minutes.

4 Heat 1 teaspoon of oil in a frying pan on a medium heat and fry the garlic and red onion for 5 minutes, until softened. Add the drained beans to the pan and cook for 2–3 minutes, then mash the beans and bake in a bowl. Leave to cool for a few minutes.

5 Place the aubergine rounds on a baking sheet, drizzle with ½ teaspoon of oil and sprinkle with sea salt. Place in the oven for 10 minutes.

6 Season the bean mix with sea salt and black pepper and mix in half the balsamic vinegar. Form into 4 burger shapes. Heat ½ tablespoon of oil in the same frying pan on a medium heat and fry the bean burgers for 4–5 minutes each side, until golden brown.

7 Peel and de-stone the avocado and crush in a bowl with a fork.

8 Serve each bean burger with a spoonful of avocado on top and place in between two aubergine slices (to act as a bun). Serve with the rocket, scattered with the roasted beetroot and sunflower seeds and drizzled with the remaining balsamic vinegar.

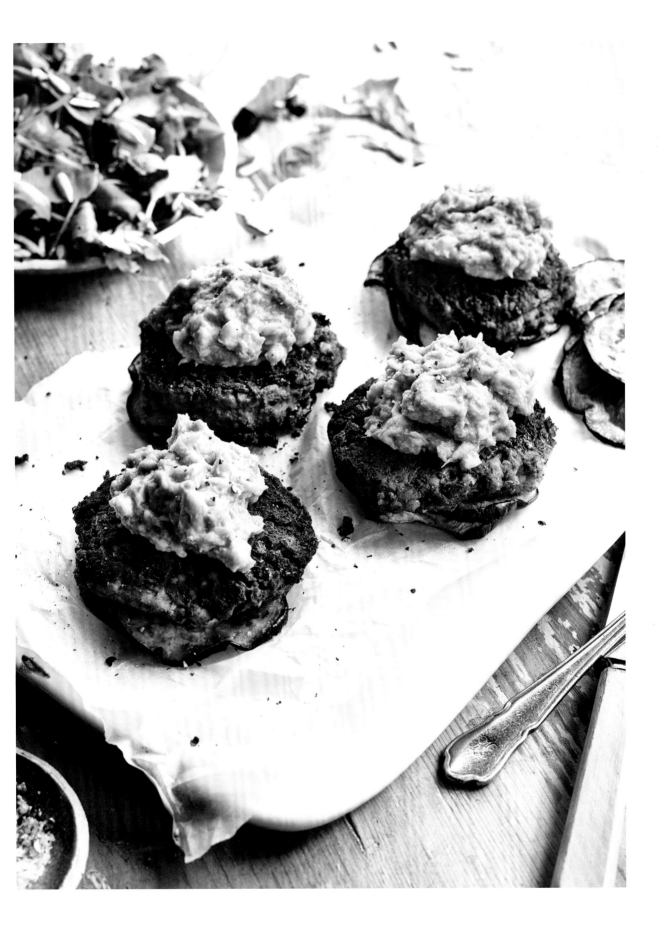

The glistening black beluga lentils, so-called because they look similar to caviar, are usually slightly more expensive than the common green or brown varieties, but we think they work better in these veggie burgers as they hold their shape when cooked.

SWEET POTATO, LENTIL & AVOCADO BURGERS WITH BAKED PORTOBELLO

300g sweet potatoes
2 garlic cloves
2 portobello mushrooms
coconut or olive oil
4 spring onions
1 avocado
120g drained tinned black
   beluga lentils
1 tsp smoked paprika
2 tbsp coconut flour
40g rocket
juice of 1 lemon
sea salt and black pepper

1 Preheat the oven to 180°C/gas mark 4.

2 Peel the sweet potatoes and chop into 1cm pieces. Place in a saucepan, cover with boiling water and add a pinch of sea salt. Simmer for 10 minutes, until softened.

3 Meanwhile, finely chop the garlic and remove the stalk from the portobello mushrooms. Place the mushrooms on a baking tray and sprinkle over the garlic and a pinch of sea salt. Drizzle over ½ tablespoon of oil and bake in the oven for 10–15 minutes.

4 Finely slice the spring onions. Peel and de-stone the avocado and slice thinly.

5 Drain and mash the sweet potatoes. Mix the black beluga lentils with the sweet potato, spring onions and smoked paprika. Season with sea salt and black pepper. Form the mixture into 4 burgers and dust with the coconut flour.

6 Heat ½ tablespoon of oil in a frying pan and fry the sweet potato and lentil burgers for 3–4 minutes each side, until golden brown.

7 To serve, place the sweet potato and lentil burgers on a plate and layer over the sliced avocado. Serve alongside the baked portobello mushrooms and the rocket and drizzle over the lemon juice.

This lightly fried plaice, a popular flat fish, is topped with a sprinkling of crispy capers and served alongside British asparagus, in season in the UK from May to early July, when there is usually an abundance. We've infused the accompanying quinoa with the lovely anise-flavoured dill for an excellent dose of vitamins A and C, which protect the body against free radicals.

PAN-FRIED PLAICE WITH ASPARAGUS, DILL QUINOA & CRISPY CAPERS

80g quinoa
300ml boiling water
140g cherry tomatoes
1 leek
140g asparagus
handful of fresh dill
coconut oil or olive oil
20g capers
2 x 150g plaice fillets
juice of 1 lemon
sea salt and black pepper

1 Preheat the oven to 180°C/gas mark 4.

2 Rinse the quinoa and place it in a saucepan with the boiling water and a pinch of sea salt. Simmer for 15 minutes.

3 Slice the cherry tomatoes in half and thinly slice the leek, removing the root end. Trim the asparagus and finely chop the dill. Place the leek and asparagus on a baking tray, drizzle with 2 teaspoons of oil and roast in the oven for 10–15 minutes.

4 Meanwhile, heat 1 teaspoon of oil in a frying pan and fry the capers over a medium-high heat for 4–5 minutes, until turning crispy. Remove from the pan and keep warm.

5 Season the plaice with sea salt and black pepper. Heat ½ tablespoon of oil in the same frying pan and fry the fish for 2–3 minutes each side, until cooked through.

6 Mix ½ tablespoon of olive oil with half the lemon juice and a quarter of the chopped dill to make a lemon dill sauce.

7 Drain the quinoa and stir through the rest of the dill and lemon juice. Add the cherry tomatoes and roasted leeks and mix well.

8 To serve, carefully place the fish on plates, drizzle over the lemon dill sauce and sprinkle over the crispy capers. Serve with the dill quinoa and asparagus.

We make our own zingy salsa verde by chopping capers, vitamin-packed fresh parsley and basil and mixing them with lemon juice and olive oil – a perfect partner to delicate white fish like sea bass. Millet, highly nutritious and gluten free, is one of the least allergenic grains around, and contains tryptophan, an amino acid which generates serotonin to help balance mood and regulate sleep. Just make sure you toast the millet grains for a couple of minutes in a dry pan before adding the water, to help them hold their shape.

PAN-FRIED SEA BASS WITH SALSA VERDE & ROASTED TOMATO MILLET

80g millet
400ml boiling water
1 red pepper
120g cherry tomatoes
olive oil
handful of fresh basil
handful of fresh flat-leaf parsley
2 garlic cloves
2 tsp capers
juice of 1 lemon
2 x 150g sea bass fillets
sea salt and black pepper

1 Preheat the oven to 200°C/gas mark 6.

2 Heat a dry saucepan, then pour in the millet and toast it for 2 minutes, stirring constantly. Pour in the boiling water, reduce the heat, cover the pan and cook for 15 minutes.

3 Meanwhile, chop the red pepper into 2cm pieces and slice the cherry tomatoes in half. Place the pepper and tomatoes on a baking tray, sprinkle over a pinch of sea salt and drizzle over ½ tablespoon of oil. Roast in the oven for 10–15 minutes.

4 To make the salsa verde, finely chop the basil and parsley leaves. Finely chop the garlic and roughly chop the capers. Put the basil, parsley, garlic and capers into a bowl with half the lemon juice and ½ tablespoon of olive oil. Season and mix well.

5 Heat ½ tablespoon of oil in a frying pan. Season the sea bass fillets with sea salt and black pepper, place in the pan skin side down and fry for 2–3 minutes each side, until cooked through.

6 Drain the millet and stir in the rest of the lemon juice and the roasted peppers and tomatoes. Season with sea salt and black pepper.

7 To serve, place the roasted pepper and tomato millet on warm plates, top with the sea bass fillets, and spoon over the salsa verde.

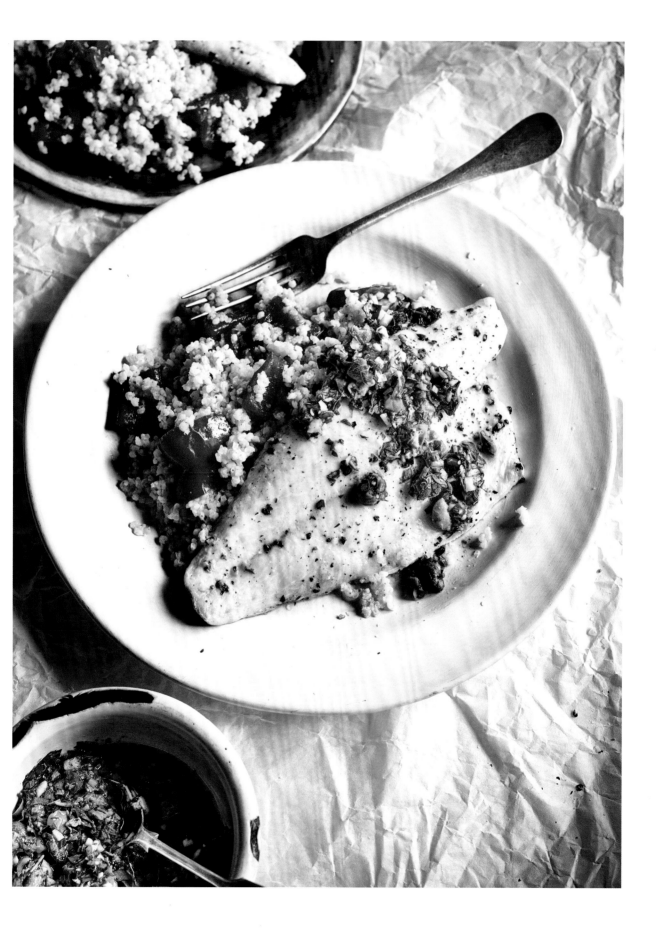

One of our favourite recipes, this is our healthy take on fried chicken – protein-packed and really simple to make. We coat sliced chicken breast in egg, ground almonds and spices and bake it until crisp. We've used the less common purple variety of sweet potato for our fries, not only for its vibrant colour, but also because it is loaded with anthocyanin pigment for protecting the gut, but you could use ordinary sweet potatoes if you can't source purple ones.

CRISPY CHICKEN WITH PURPLE SWEET POTATO FRIES & AVOCADO SALSA

250g purple sweet potatoes
coconut or olive oil
2 x 170g chicken breasts
8 tbsp ground almonds
1 tsp smoked paprika
½ tsp chilli powder
1 egg
1 avocado
120g cherry tomatoes
handful of fresh coriander
juice of 1 lime
sea salt and black pepper

1 Preheat the oven to 200°C/gas mark 6.

2 Peel the sweet potatoes and cut them into fries, then place on a baking tray and drizzle over ½ tablespoon of oil and a pinch of salt.

3 Slice the chicken into thin strips.

4 In a bowl, mix the ground almonds with the smoked paprika, chilli powder and a generous pinch of sea salt. Crack the egg into a separate bowl and whisk with a fork.

5 Dip each strip of chicken into the egg and then into the spiced ground almond mix. Place the chicken strips on a second baking tray, lined with a sheet of baking paper (or spread with ½ tablespoon of oil), and bake in the oven for 20 minutes, turning halfway, until golden and cooked through.

6 At the same time, place the tray of sweet potato fries in the oven for 20 minutes, turning halfway through.

7 Meanwhile peel and de-stone the avocado, cut the cherry tomatoes in half and finely chop the coriander. In a bowl, roughly crush the avocado with a fork and mix with the tomatoes, coriander and lime juice. Season with salt and pepper.

8 Place the crispy chicken strips on plates, alongside the purple sweet potato fries and avocado salsa. Drizzle over the rest of the lime juice.

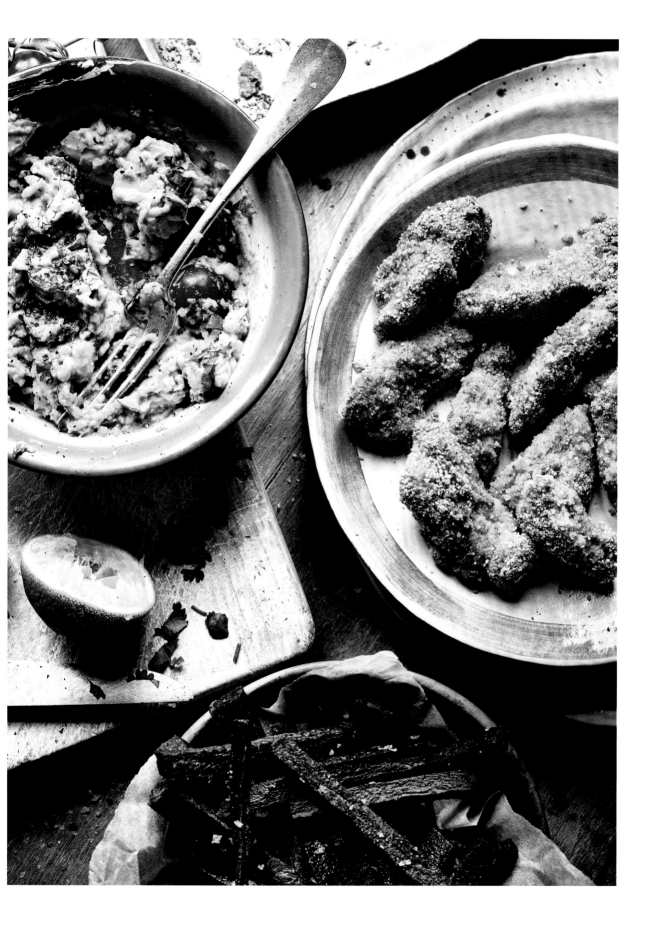

This is a lovely dish to eat al fresco on a warm summer's evening. Baking chicken with pomegranate molasses gives it a sweet, tangy flavour that is a perfect foil for the slight bitterness of chicory. We've used red chicory for its colour (but you could use white chicory instead) and paired it with roasted British asparagus and juicy orange segments, packed with vitamin C to prevent summer colds and flu.

POMEGRANATE CHICKEN WITH ASPARAGUS, CHICORY, ORANGE & WALNUTS

2 x 170g chicken breasts
olive oil
2 tbsp pomegranate molasses
80g buckwheat
400ml boiling water
1 head of chicory
140g asparagus
1 orange
30g walnuts
sea salt and black pepper

1 Preheat the oven to 200°C/gas mark 6.

2 Place the chicken breasts on a baking tray and season with sea salt and black pepper. In a bowl mix ½ tablespoon of oil and half the pomegranate molasses and spoon over the chicken. Place in the oven for 25 minutes, or until the chicken is cooked through.

3 Meanwhile, rinse the buckwheat, place in a saucepan with the boiling water and simmer for 15 minutes.

4 Slice the end off the chicory and cut in half, then slice each half lengthways into 4 pieces. Trim the asparagus. Place the chicory and asparagus on a baking tray, drizzle with 1 teaspoon of oil and place in the oven for 10 minutes.

5 To make the pomegranate dressing, mix the remaining pomegranate molasses with 1 tablespoon of olive oil and season with salt and pepper.

6 Peel the orange and slice into segments. Roughly chop the walnuts. Slice the cooked chicken in half widthways and drain the buckwheat.

7 To serve, spoon the buckwheat on to warm plates and arrange the orange segments, chicory and asparagus over the top, followed by the chicken pieces, slightly overlapping. Drizzle over the pomegranate dressing and sprinkle over the walnuts.

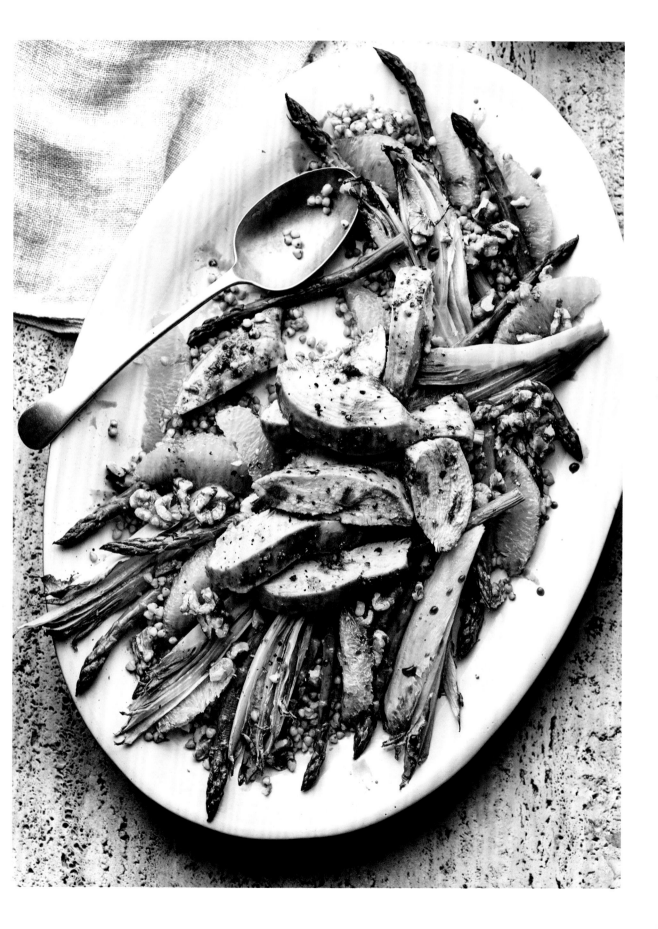

This is a lovely spring roast chicken recipe for a quick and super tasty meal. We've used chicken thighs, as they are so juicy when baked and really take on the flavour of the thyme and lemon. We've roasted baby carrots alongside the chicken and served them with steamed greens, full of vitamin K for bone strength.

LEMON & THYME CHICKEN THIGHS WITH BABY CARROTS & BUCKWHEAT

2 lemons
4 garlic cloves
200g baby carrots
300g chicken thighs, skinless and
   boneless
coconut oil or olive oil
2 tsp Dijon mustard
handful of fresh thyme
80g buckwheat
400ml boiling water
200g spring greens
sea salt and black pepper

1 Preheat the oven to 200°C / gas mark 6.

2 Cut 1 lemon into slices, then peel the garlic cloves and cut in half. Trim the carrots and slice in half lengthways.

3 Season the chicken thighs. Heat 1 teaspoon of oil in a frying pan on a medium-high heat and brown the chicken for 2–3 minutes on each side. Add the garlic cloves to the pan to brown for the last 2 minutes.

4 In a bowl, mix the mustard with half of the juice of the remaining lemon and ½ tablespoon of oil.

5 Place the chicken in an ovenproof dish with the carrots and garlic, pour over the lemon mustard sauce and place 1 or 2 lemon slices on each chicken thigh. Scatter over the thyme leaves. Bake in the oven for 15–20 minutes, or until the chicken is cooked through and the juices run clear.

6 Meanwhile, rinse the buckwheat, place in a saucepan with the boiling water and simmer for 15 minutes. Drain and stir in the remaining lemon juice. Season with salt and pepper.

7 Thinly slice the spring greens. Place them in a steamer over a pan of boiling water and steam for 6 minutes, until cooked.

8 Spoon the buckwheat on to plates and top with the chicken thighs and the juices from the pan. Serve alongside the carrots, roasted garlic and spring greens.

Chestnut mushrooms accompany the tender pork loin – these have a high water content, so are low in calories, but support immune function. Nutrient-dense broccoli 'rice', simply grated raw and cooked with a little water for a few minutes, is a quick and nourishing replacement to white rice.

COCONUT & PAPRIKA PORK STROGANOFF WITH BROCCOLI RICE

1 red onion
160g chestnut mushrooms
2 garlic cloves
handful of fresh flat-leaf parsley
2 x 150g pork loin steaks
coconut or olive oil
2 tsp smoked paprika
200ml coconut milk
1 tsp wholegrain mustard
juice of 1 lemon
1 head of broccoli
sea salt and black pepper

1 Finely slice the red onion and chestnut mushrooms and finely chop the garlic and parsley. Slice the pork into thin strips.

2 Heat 1 teaspoon of oil in a medium-sized pan over a medium heat and fry the onion and garlic for 3 minutes.

3 Add the sliced pork and cook for 5 minutes, until golden. Add the mushrooms and smoked paprika and cook for 3 minutes.

4 Add the coconut milk and wholegrain mustard and season with salt and black pepper. Simmer for 10 minutes, until the pork is cooked through. Stir in half the lemon juice, to taste.

5 Meanwhile, to make the broccoli rice, grate the broccoli to a rice consistency. Put the broccoli rice into a saucepan on a medium heat with 2 tablespoons of water, the remaining lemon juice and a pinch of sea salt. Stir continuously for 4 minutes, until the broccoli is tender.

6 Mix half the chopped parsley through the broccoli rice and serve on warm plates, topped with the pork stroganoff and sprinkled with the remaining chopped parsley.

We hope you love these fragrant pork meatballs as much as we do. Infused with Thai flavours and nestled in a creamy, nourishing courgette noodle soup, this is comfort in a mouthful. Fresh lemongrass, ginger, red chilli and Thai basil pack a punchy flavour and bring the soup to life.

THAI PORK MEATBALLS IN A COCONUT & COURGETTI NOODLE SOUP

1 red pepper
120g chestnut mushrooms
280g courgettes
4cm fresh ginger
1 fresh lemongrass stalk
1 fresh red chilli
handful of fresh Thai basil
300g pork mince
1 vegetable stock cube
200ml boiling water
200ml coconut milk
juice of 1 lime
sea salt and black pepper

1 Finely slice the red pepper and the mushrooms. Remove the ends of the courgettes, but leave the skin on. Prepare the courgette noodles using a peeler and slice the courgette into long thin strips (or use a julienne peeler or spiraliser, if you have one).

2 Peel and finely chop the ginger. Trim the end of the lemongrass, remove the outer layer and finely chop. Finely chop the red chilli and roughly chop half the Thai basil.

3 Mix the ginger, lemongrass, chilli and basil in a bowl with the pork mince and season with salt and pepper. Form into 16 small balls.

4 Heat 1 tablespoon of oil in a medium-sized pan and fry the pork meatballs for 15 minutes, turning frequently, until golden brown and cooked through.

5 Meanwhile, dissolve the vegetable stock cube in the boiling water and put into a saucepan with the coconut milk.

6 Bring to the boil, add the red pepper, mushrooms and courgette noodles and simmer for 3 minutes.

7 Spoon the coconut soup and vegetables into a bowl and top with the meatballs, the remaining Thai basil leaves and the lime juice. Enjoy!

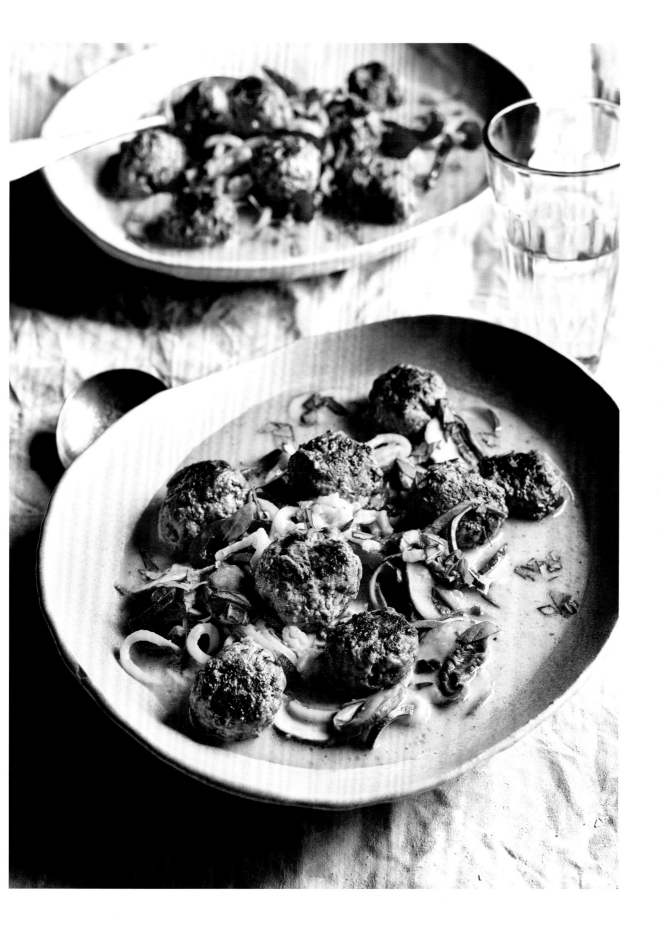

Pink peppercorns are deliciously sweet dried berries with a light peppery flavour – we crush these and rub them on to steaks for a flavour-packed seasoning. We like to use seasonal vegetables like kohlrabi, which we've made into tasty chips. Kohlrabi is a member of the brassica family, along with kale, cabbage and radishes, and has a delicate turnip flavour. It is in season from June to November in the UK and can be found in specialist grocery shops and markets, but if you can't find it, celeriac works well in its place.

PINK PEPPERCORN STEAK WITH KOHLRABI CHIPS & CREAMY GARLIC MUSHROOMS

2 garlic cloves
120g chestnut mushrooms
½ red shallot
1 tbsp apple cider vinegar
olive oil
2 tsp pink peppercorns
2 x 170g sirloin steaks
1 kohlrabi
handful of fresh thyme
20g creamed coconut
50ml boiling water
40g lamb's lettuce
sea salt and black pepper

1 Preheat the oven to 200°C/gas mark 6.

2 Finely chop or crush the garlic and thinly slice the mushrooms.

3 Finely dice the shallot and place in a bowl with the apple cider vinegar and ½ tablespoon of oil.

4 In a pestle and mortar (or using a rolling pin), crush the pink peppercorns and mix with a pinch of salt and pepper and ½ tablespoon of oil. Rub on to the steaks and set aside.

5 Peel the kohlrabi and slice into thin chips. Mix with a pinch of salt, ½ tablespoon of oil and the thyme leaves. Spread the chips out on a baking tray and cook in the oven for 20 minutes, turning halfway.

6 Heat a griddle pan. Cook the steaks until golden brown, 2–3 minutes each side for medium rare or 4–5 minutes each side for well done. Remove from the pan and leave to rest.

7 Dissolve the creamed coconut in the boiling water. Heat ½ tablespoon of oil in a frying pan on a medium heat and add the garlic and mushrooms. Fry for 3 minutes, then add the coconut and cook for 2 minutes. Season.

8 Arrange the steaks on warm plates with the mushrooms spooned over and serve with the chips and the lamb's lettuce drizzled with the shallot dressing.

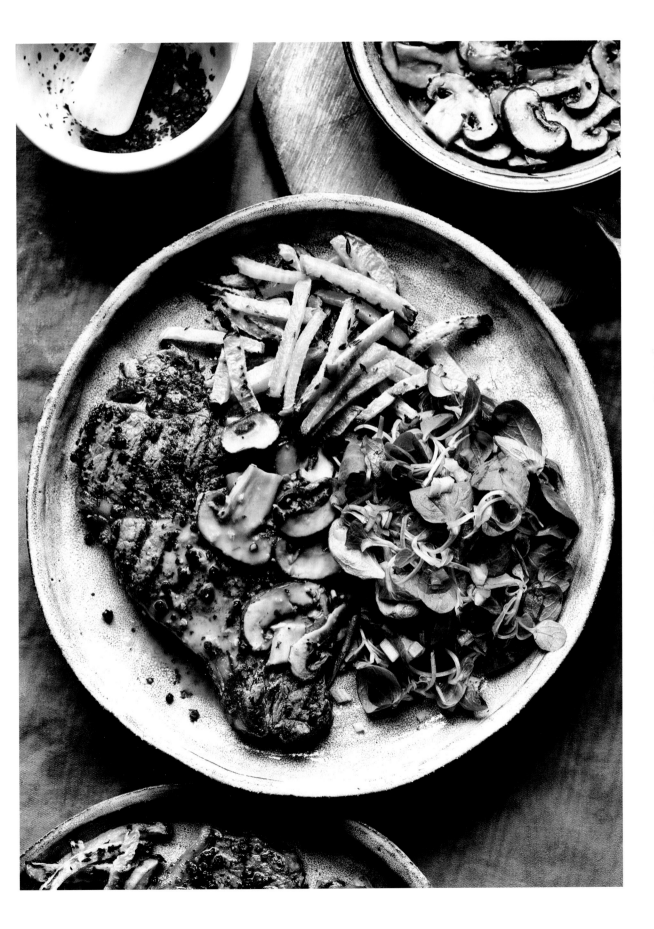

This juicy beef and mustard burger sits on an oven-baked portobello mushroom, another nutritious and flavour-packed alternative to a burger bun. The baked carrot fries are sprinkled with fresh rosemary as its fragrant flavour pairs beautifully with the sweetness of the carrots. Rosemary is one of the most effective herbs at reducing inflammation, while its oils have been known to improve cognitive ability, even enhancing concentration and memory.

BEEF & MUSTARD BURGER WITH BALSAMIC ONIONS & ROSEMARY CARROT FRIES

2 portobello mushrooms
1 red onion
3 sprigs of fresh rosemary
300g carrots
coconut or olive oil
300g beef mince
2 tsp wholegrain mustard
1½ tbsp balsamic vinegar
1 avocado
40g rocket
sea salt and black pepper

1 Preheat the oven to 200°C/gas mark 6.

2 Remove the stalks from the portobello mushrooms and finely slice the red onion.

3 Finely chop the rosemary (removing the stalk). Peel the carrots and cut into fries, then place on a baking tray and sprinkle over a pinch of sea salt, the rosemary and ½ tablespoon of oil. Bake in the oven for 20–25 minutes, until the carrots start to become golden. Halfway through, turn them over, then sit the mushrooms next to them. Put the tray back into the oven for the remainder of the cooking time.

4 Place the beef mince and mustard in a bowl, season and mix well. Shape into 2 burgers, place on a baking tray and bake in the oven for 10–15 minutes, until turning golden and cooked through.

5 Meanwhile, heat 1 teaspoon of oil in a pan on a medium heat and add the red onion. Cook for 10 minutes, until softened and golden brown, then add half the balsamic vinegar and cook for a further 5 minutes.

6 Peel and de-stone the avocado, then place in a bowl and crush with the back of a fork.

7 To serve, place a mushroom on each plate, top each one with a burger, then add the crushed avocado, followed by the balsamic onions. Serve alongside the carrot fries and the rocket, drizzled with the remaining balsamic vinegar.

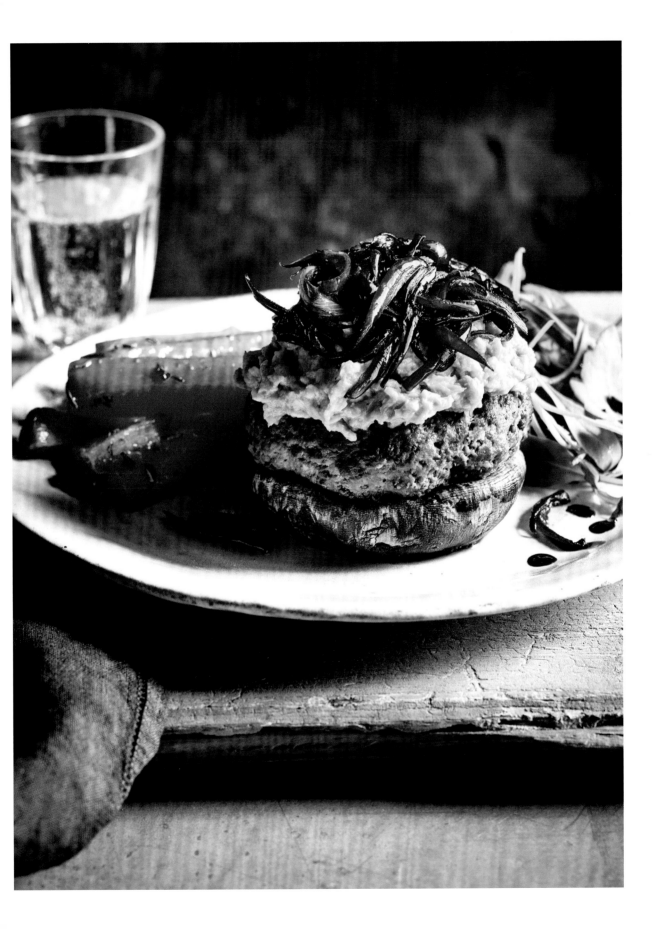

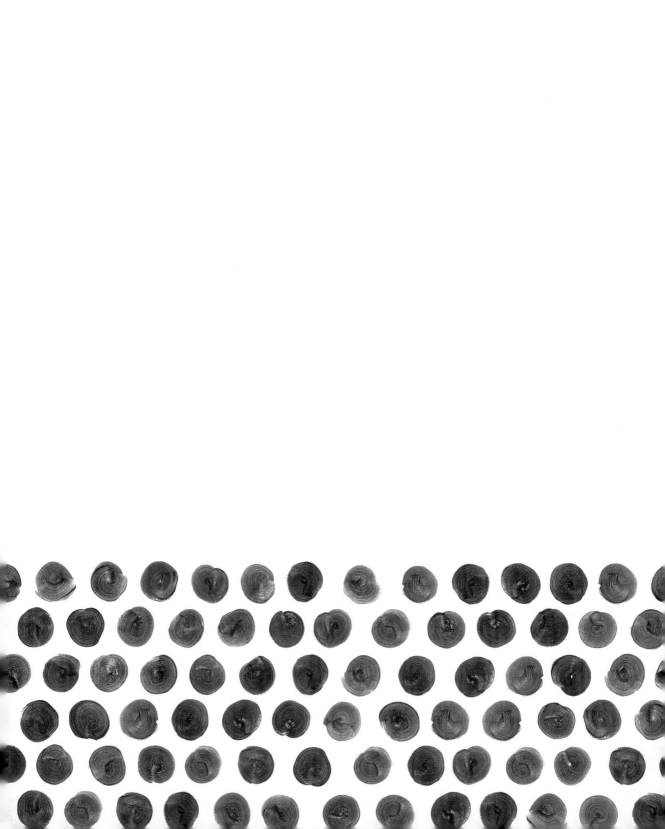

SNACKS
+
SWEET TREATS

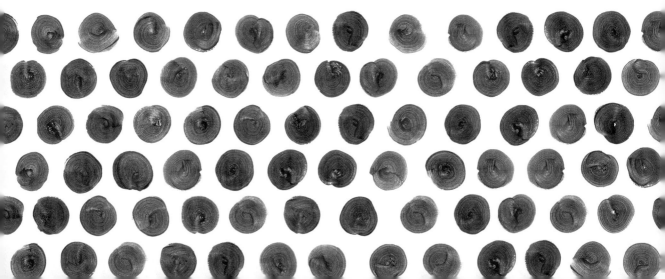

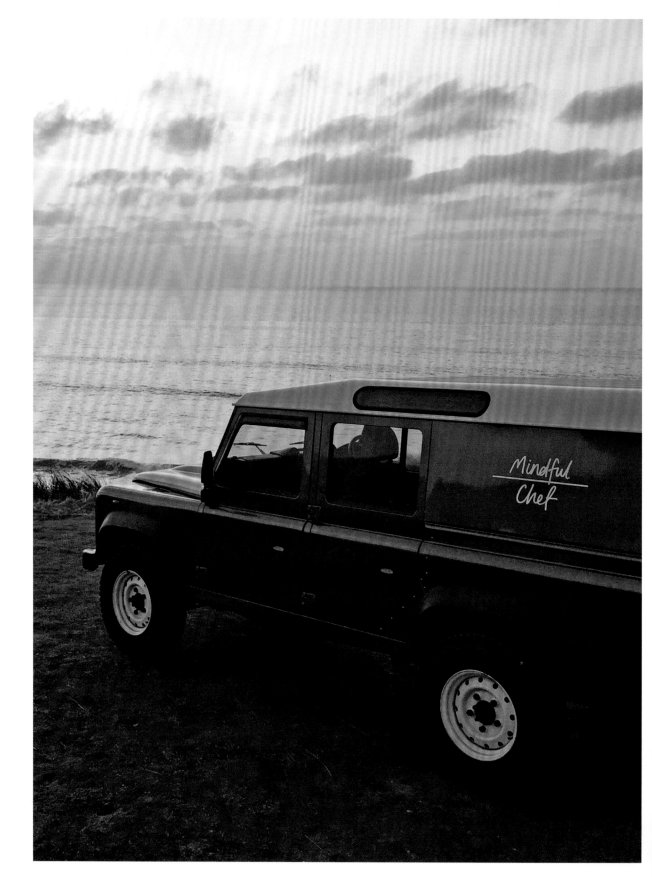

SNACKS + SWEET TREATS

As I've got older and have became more interested in the effects of nutrition on our bodies, I've lost the interest I had in sweet things as a child. I haven't cut treats out completely, and will never say no to a piece of good-quality dark chocolate, but I very rarely shop for desserts or have any in my fridge.

Generally my snacks tend to be made up of smaller meals trying to hit all of the essential food groups – protein, carbohydrates and fats. However, every now and then I crave food that is a bit indulgent. This section has some of our favourite sweet treats like black bean brownies, energy-boosting protein balls or delicious matcha and cashew cookies, all of which can be enjoyed as a pause with a hot drink on the go. These snacks work really well to take to work or on long trips (I can't tell you how many times protein balls have stopped me from reaching for unhealthy, tasteless travel snacks). We've also included our strawberry and coconut banana ice cream, which is my personal favourite for chilling out on a Sunday evening watching a film. Eating tasty snacks full of real, good-for-you ingredients means that you'll be eating food that not only you love but your body will love too.

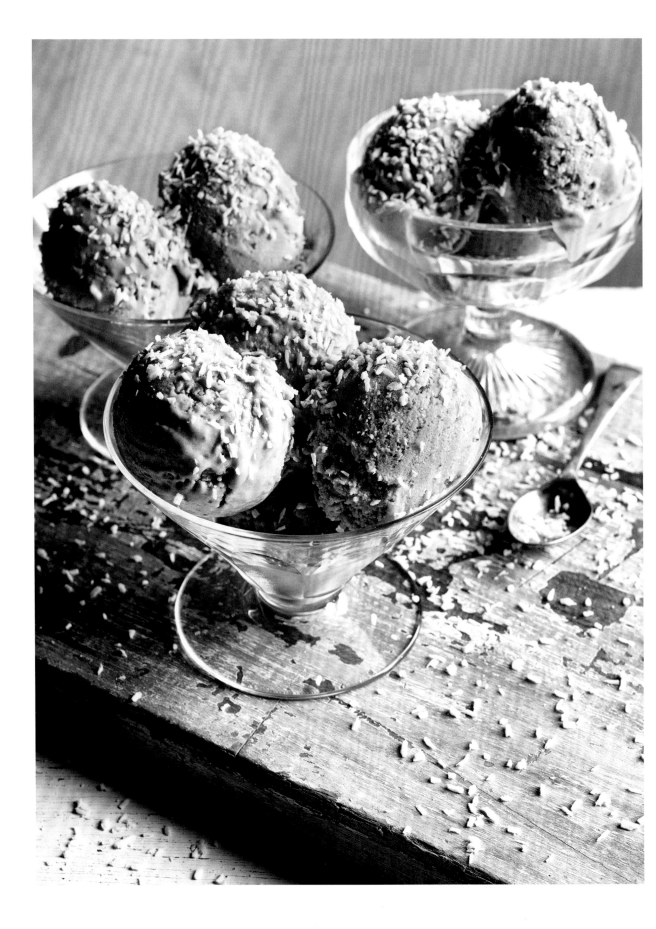

Instead of reaching for shop-bought ice cream, try making this incredible-tasting natural version yourself. It's such a simple and quick recipe with only four ingredients. You just need to freeze the bananas and strawberries for a few hours (or overnight) and after that it takes only 5 minutes to make. You'll be amazed at the smooth creamy texture. Get creative and try variations, such as chocolate and peanut, made by substituting the strawberries with a tablespoon of raw cacao, a tablespoon of peanut butter and a teaspoon of maple syrup.

STRAWBERRY & COCONUT BANANA ICE CREAM

2 frozen bananas, peeled and each cut into 3 pieces

4 frozen strawberries, green stalks removed

50ml coconut milk

½ tbsp desiccated coconut

1 Place the bananas, strawberries and coconut milk in a blender or food processor and blend for 1 minute, or until all the ingredients are well combined.

2 Spoon into bowls and sprinkle over the desiccated coconut.

These decadent mouthfuls are packed with raw cacao – unprocessed cocoa powder made by cold-pressing cocoa beans that haven't been roasted and therefore contain a higher amount of beneficial antioxidant properties. Coupled with the black beans, our brownies are bursting with minerals and fibre. We've slathered them in a creamy nut butter topping; double the quantity for an extra thick layer! We're not going to pretend that these brownies aren't high in calories, but, unlike shop-bought versions, they contain a good serving of protein, and no unrefined flours or sugar, so they won't give you that energy crash after eating them.

BLACK BEAN BROWNIES WITH MAPLE NUT BUTTER

Makes 16

Brownies
480g drained and rinsed
    black beans
100g raw cacao
3 tbsp almond butter
4 eggs
250g coconut oil (in liquid form
    – you may have to heat it
    gently until it turns liquid)
200ml maple syrup
2 tsp vanilla extract
pinch of sea salt
80g cashew nuts
3 tbsp raw cacao nibs (optional)

Topping
3 tbsp maple syrup
15g raw cacao
5 tbsp cashew nut butter or
    almond butter
3–4 tbsp almond milk
1 tsp vanilla extract
2 tbsp pomegranate seeds

1 Preheat the oven to 180°C/gas mark 4.

2 Line a medium-sized baking tin (around 25 x 20cm) with baking paper and grease with coconut oil.

3 Put the black beans, raw cacao, almond butter and eggs into a food processor and blend until smooth. Add the coconut oil, maple syrup, vanilla extract and salt and blend again until combined.

4 Roughly chop the cashew nuts and stir into the mix along with the raw cacao nibs, if using.

5 Pour the black bean brownie mix into the lined baking tin, then bake for 25 minutes. You can increase the cooking time if you prefer, but we like ours to have a fudgy texture. Remove and leave to cool.

6 Meanwhile, make the maple nut butter topping. Put the maple syrup, raw cacao, nut butter, almond milk and vanilla extract into a food processor and blend until smooth.

7 Once the brownies have cooled, spoon over the maple nut butter topping and sprinkle over the pomegranate seeds.

We all love an indulgent creamy salted caramel, but our version is virtually guilt-free. Instead of using high-fat butter and refined sugar, we blend dates and cashew butter to provide you with a longer-lasting release of energy. These caramels are drizzled in homemade raw chocolate – if you have any left over, try making chocolate bark. Simply pour the chocolate on to a clean chopping board lined with baking paper and sprinkle over any nuts, seeds and chopped dried fruit you have in your cupboard. Place in the fridge for 30 minutes to harden. It also makes a great gift!

SALTED CARAMEL RAW CHOCOLATES

Makes 15

Salted caramel
150g soft dates
2 tbsp cashew nut butter
2 tbsp maple syrup
generous pinch of sea salt (to taste)

Raw chocolate
50g raw cacao butter
3 tbsp raw cacao powder
1½ tbsp maple syrup
pinch of sea salt

1 To make the salted caramel, first roughly chop the dates and blend in a food processor for 1 minute, until smooth. Add the cashew nut butter and maple syrup and blend again until fully combined. Then add 2 tablespoons of cold water and the salt and blend for 30 seconds.

2 Transfer the salted caramel date mixture to a bowl. Place heaped teaspoons of the mixture on a plate or board lined with baking paper, until the mixture is all used up. Cover with cling film and place in the freezer for 20 minutes.

3 Meanwhile, make the raw chocolate to coat the caramels. Place the cacao butter in a bowl over a pan filled with gently simmering water (a bain-marie) and allow to melt gently. Once melted, use a hand whisk to mix in the raw cacao followed by the maple syrup and salt. Whisk to combine, then remove from the heat. Leave to cool for a few minutes, so the chocolate thickens slightly.

4 Meanwhile, take the caramels out of the freezer. Roll each spoonful into a ball in your hands and place on a fresh piece of baking paper. Spoon or pour over the raw chocolate and leave to set in the fridge for 15 minutes.

Our delicious cookies are packed with health-boosting superfoods and are so easy to make. Matcha is a Japanese green tea that uses the whole green tea leaf ground into a fine powder and contains much higher level of antioxidants than other green teas. We've combined it with creamy cashew nut butter, a great source of protein, minerals and vitamin C. When buying nut butters, check the ingredients to make sure that there are no added oils – the best quality nut butters are made solely of nuts.

MATCHA & CASHEW COOKIES

Makes 10

270g crunchy cashew nut butter
100g coconut palm sugar
1 tsp bicarbonate of soda
1 egg
1 tbsp matcha powder
40g cashew nuts, roughly
   chopped

1 Preheat the oven to 180°C/gas mark 4.

2 Put the cashew nut butter, coconut palm sugar and bicarbonate of soda into a bowl and mix together until combined, then beat in the egg to form a dough. Add the matcha powder and stir well, then stir in the chopped cashew nuts.

3 Form the cookie dough into 10 balls and place them on a baking tray lined with baking paper.

4 Flatten the balls with the palm of your hand to form a cookie shape (they will expand a bit when cooking).

5 Bake in the oven for 8–10 minutes, until lightly golden brown. Leave to cool for a few minutes, then place on a wire rack to cool and enjoy!

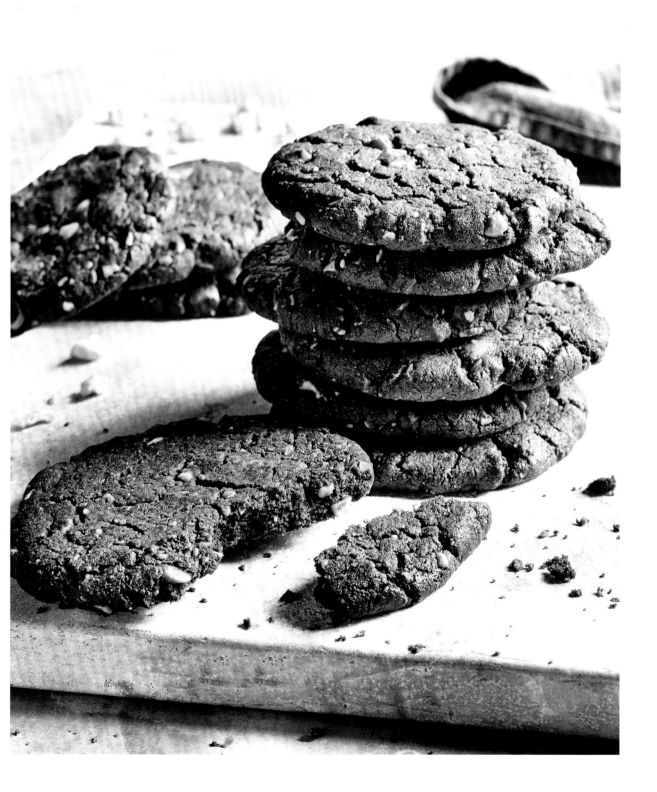

So delicious and simple to make, these energy balls are packed full of protein, vitamins and omega-3 fatty acids from the ground flaxseed, chia seeds, almond butter and chopped cashews. Vegan and gluten-free, they also contain the ancient superfood maca, a nutrient-dense root from South America known to boost energy and mood. The perfect afternoon pick me up... Just try not to eat them all at once!

ENERGY-BOOSTING PROTEIN BALLS

Makes 10

120g almond butter
50g ground flaxseed
2 tbsp maca powder
1 tbsp chia seeds
1 tbsp desiccated coconut
1 tbsp maple syrup

To coat
15g cashew nuts, finely chopped

1 Mix all the ingredients together in a bowl until fully combined, then form into 10 small balls.

2 Put the finely chopped cashew nuts on a plate and roll the balls over them until evenly coated.

3 Place in the fridge for 30 minutes, to firm up.

INDEX

Our biggest thank you must go to Rob, without whom Mindful Chef would never have become a reality. The last two years have been the most amazing journey and it's been a lot of fun sharing it with you.

Louisa, thank you for teaching us so much about food and cooking. This book is testament to your amazing abilities as a chef. Not only did we gain a fantastic chef but also a dear friend. Thank you for helping us make Mindful Chef so successful.

A big thank you to Ben, Sam and the rest of the team at Penguin Random House. Your enthusiasm and belief in Mindful Chef has made writing this book so enjoyable. Thank you for helping us spread our message.

To the wonderful team that helped put this book together. Thank you Imogen for all of your hard work and for putting up with us while we wrote the book. To Nikki, Kris, Kat and Louie we are eternally grateful – you managed to bring our story and our food to life and the book looks stunning.

To Lydia Hardwick for the loan of her plates for the photography.

To our customers and the whole Mindful Chef community. Thank you for your support and overwhelming belief in Mindful Chef and our mission to make healthy eating easy. We can't quite believe how far we have come and would never have dreamed of writing a book after such a short period of time.

To the Mindful Chef team who make every day a lot of fun. We are very lucky to be able to work with such a talented group of people who share our beliefs. Your energy and passion for Mindful Chef and all your work are fantastic.

To our families for their unwavering support, not only with the book but also in believing in Mindful Chef from the start. Through the good times and the bad you have always been there for us and we couldn't have done this without you. Thank you!

To Claudia for always being there. Through the endless ramblings and late nights spent proofreading you never hesitated to help. Thank you.

FOLLOW MINDFUL CHEF

 www.instagram.com/mindfulchefuk

 www.facebook.com/MindfulChefUK

 @MindfulChefUK

www.mindfulchef.com

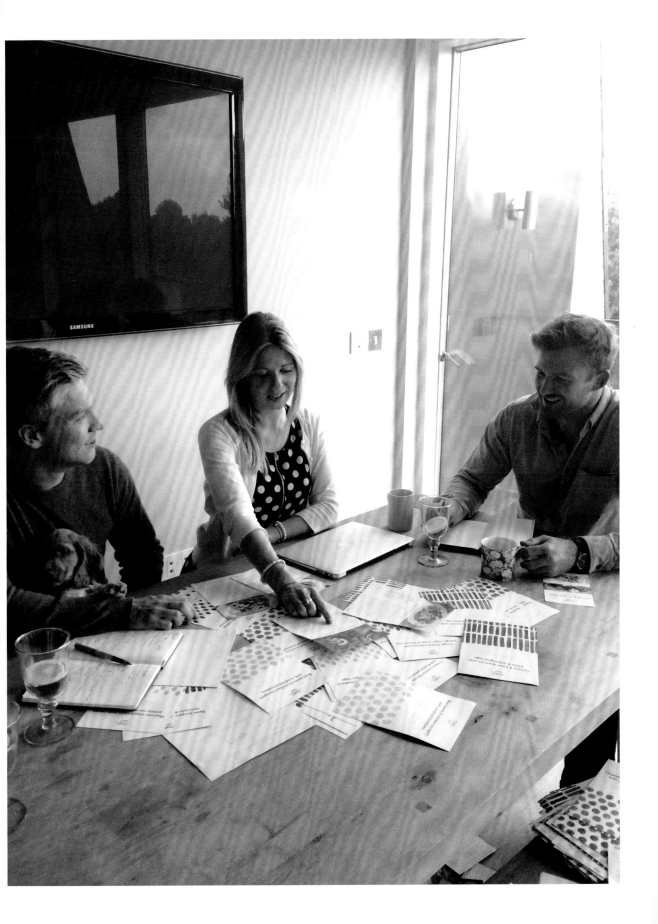

1 3 5 7 9 10 8 6 4 2

Century
20 Vauxhall Bridge Road
London SW1V 2SA

Century is part of the Penguin Random House group of companies whose addresses can be found at global.
penguinrandomhouse.com.

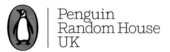

First published by Century in 2017

www.penguin.co.uk

A CIP catalogue record for this book is available from the British Library.

ISBN 9781780896694

Printed and bound in China by C&C Offset Printing Co., Ltd

Penguin Random House is committed to a sustainable future for our business, our readers and our planet.
This book is made from Forest Stewardship Council® certified paper.

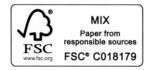

Design: nicandlou.com
Recipe photography: Kris Kirkham
Reportage photography: Mindful Chef
Editor: Imogen Fortes
Food styling: Kat Mead
Prop styling: Louie Waller